THE YOGA OF LIGHT

THE YOGA OF LIGHT

Hatha Yoga Pradipika
India's Classical Handbook

HANS-ULRICH RIEKER

Translated by Elsy Becherer

HERDER AND HERDER

1971
HERDER AND HERDER NEW YORK
232 Madison Avenue, New York 10016

ISBN 665-00000-6
Library of Congress Catalog Card Number: 79–167868
© 1971 by Herder and Herder, Inc.
Manufactured in the United States

CONTENTS

TRANSLATOR'S NOTE

In Indian philosophy it is generally understood that hatha yoga is one distinct path to liberation and raja yoga another. *Hatha Yoga Pradipika* shows a rare and fruitful combination of the two paths: hatha and raja.

The slokas of this ancient classical text are presented in an extremely terse and often highly symbolic language, which makes them practically unintelligible without commentary. It is therefore very fortunate that Hans-Ulrich Rieker has given us in his commentaries the benefit of his experiences and knowledge acquired in the course of many years of intensive training with native teachers. He is a highly accomplished yogi but is always aware of the Western student's problems. Thus his translation and commentaries make *Hatha Yoga Pradipika* truly a vade mecum for the serious student of yoga.

This is a faithful translation of the original German text, *Das klassische Yoga-Lehrbuch Indiens*. It is complete with all the valuable and elucidating commentaries except for a few passages of philosophical exegesis, and some comparative references to Goethe's *Faust,* which would be of little or no interest to modern English and American readers. Within the classical text passages, interpolations inserted by Hans-Ulrich Rieker have been set off in brackets, while additional interpolations made by the present translator for the sake of clarity have been set in roman type within brackets. Finally, an extensive index of terms and a list of books recommended for further reading have been added to the present edition.

Questions will no doubt arise about the presentation of the slokas in a retranslation of the Sanskrit from the German into English. This objection is partly overcome by the fact that the translator not only had recourse to two early translations from Sanskrit ino English by the Indian scholars, Swami Srinvasa Iyangar and Pancham Sinh, but also is familiar with the subject and terminology through 12 years of training and practice with the Indian yogi and scholar, Dr. Rammurti S. Mishra.

I wish to thank David and Debby, whose enthusiasm and valuable suggestions constantly sustained my efforts.

E.B.

INTRODUCTION

Is it really worth while for the average reader to read a scholarly classic, a book that has been pulled off a dusty shelf and translated into a modern Western language? This question occupied my mind for a long time, until I realized to my surprise that the subjects of my research, the yogis, are anything but dry scientists. I noticed that the most successful among them were those who understood how to transform old traditions and terminologies into the spirit of the time. Similarly, I have seen more laughing yogis than smiling professors. And that encouraged me to break the dry sacred tradition and to search for living wisdom in the ancient texts. This is a serious decision. Yoga is not a trifling jest if we consider that any misunderstanding in the practice of yoga can mean death or insanity. That a misunderstood yoga can be dangerous has been proven by many a student who started his practice in grim determination rather than relaxed joy. It is not the dry letter but the pulsating life in the ancient teachings that are transmitted to us not by scholars but by the wise men.

Our endeavor here is not so much to enrich science as to enrich ourselves; and he who enriches his self, his inner Self, does he not also enrich the science of man? Yoga is the science of man and his potential. Yoga as a deadly serious business does not interest me. I want yoga to bring a deeper joy into my life. I do not wish to make anyone smarter, nor is this the endeavor of yoga. For cleverness has proven itself much less than that rare wisdom for which yoga has always stood. It is quite easy to accumulate a vast store of knowledge and still get under the wheel of fate. Real wisdom is not at all encyclopedic, but it knows how to master everyday life, and that to me seems vastly more important. Knowledge of the world beyond my horizon is of interest only after I have removed all dangers on this side. He who is interested in the manifold aspects of science and with that forgets his own self deprives himself of the experience of the greatest mystery the world has to offer. We must certainly be grateful to science for giving us so much that we so quickly take for granted. But why do we so quickly take things for granted? Because at some time or other someone puts aside the book of science and realizes its practicability through his own experiments. This book too should eventually be put aside in favor of practical experiments.

Here science has made a mysterious text available to us: the *Hatha Yoga Pradipika,* by Yoga Swami Svatmarama. And we shall try together to find hidden in the folds of this strange text the treasure that can bring us closer to the path of wisdom than is suspected by the confirmed skeptics.

In order to achieve this, it is necessary that we pretend to know as little about ourselves as a newborn babe. Of course, modern science has provided us with a fabulous amount of knowledge concerning our body and mind. But although it is possible, after years of study, to know all the secrets of the mechanism of an automobile, with the human being we will never succeed in the same way. The most important problems will never yield to theoretical probing. Love, hatred, diplomacy, control of situations, economy of forces, interest, and futility— all this is in a day's work. And who despairs just because the deepest sources of these events are unknown to us? Everything in life is simple as long as one takes everything for granted. It is when we want to know "why" that we stop in our tracks. Is it necessary to know why? If we have practically no problems, why create them theoretically? The answer would be quite clear if we really did have no problems. Unfortunately, we do have them, both with our surroundings and with ourselves. When one of these problems becomes serious we realize how imperfect we are, and the question becomes acute: must we really be content with such a full measure of imperfection, and is this imperfection man's immanent fate? We must admit that this or that person in world history was more perfect than we are but our reverence for such a person does not induce us to make him our teacher. Not *through* others do we want to become perfect, but *like* others. Nor do we want to go to the trouble of *becoming* perfect. We seek the sudden, joyful awareness that fundamentally we *are* perfect.

It is encouraging that this natural attitude is not as presumptuous as it may seem. We really do not have to adopt the wisdom of others; we have our own at our disposal. But there are certain obstacles to prevent its unfoldment. To remove these obstacles has from time immemorial been the greatest endeavor of mankind. And some actually did find ways and means: Zoroaster, the Buddha, Lao-tzu, Christ, to mention but a few. It is from them that humanity received its greatest treasures, and humanity gratefully received the gift and tried to utilize it.

But since evidently nothing is more attractive than to confound the words of great masters and present them according to one's own taste, whole libraries have grown around the teachings of the great ones, so that we are now hardly in a position to find the real words of the masters among the presumptuous "improvements." The Parsis admit that only a small fraction of their master's teachings has been preserved. Lao-tzu has been translated so ingeniously that it is possible to understand the exact contrary of what he intended to say. If the Buddha had really made all the speeches attributed to him, he would have had to speak day and night for a hundred years. And if we had understood Christ's teachings more intuitively, the world of today would be a different place. No doubt we can learn immeasurably from these great ones provided we can reach the true teachings, but that is very difficult. For one, we are at the mercy of translators who at best may be philologists, but certainly are not saints who have put into practice the teachings they are putting before us. For example, anyone who has even a casual knowledge of biblical texts will be dismayed to find passages that were completely misunderstood by such a man as Martin Luther. And it is even worse with K. E. Neumann, the great Buddha translator. His work is almost completely free of the kernels of real wisdom. Here too, the original text reveals whole new worlds.

Well, we might ask, were these people completely blind? Let us look at the dictionaries and compare. Philologically, both are right—the old translator as well as the modern critic. So either might want to take a pencil and write down his own interpretation (an improvement, no doubt) in the margins, as was done in old manuscripts.

Now let us imagine what would happen—and it happens constantly—in such languages as Chinese or Sanskrit, where one word may have twenty different meanings. What libraries of misinterpretation have grown in the course of a thousand years. And where is the ordinary faithful reader to find the truth among so many versions which all claim to be true? For—and this is important—every interpretation is in some way justified.

How does it stand with our text? The man who wrote it was an authority, a yogi of the highest achievements, as can be surmised by his name; the work itself indisputably holds first place among all classical yoga textbooks and is quoted by all those first-class teachers who have sat at the springs rather than the faucets of wisdom. Why, then, should we be satisfied with secondary material when we can go directly to the master himself?

Of course, the same question arises here as with Luther and

Neumann: Is the present translation authentic? This translation of *Hatha Yoga Pradipika* and my commentary on it were not done at a desk, but were, so to speak, written on my knee, on the straw mats of India. If a question arose and my own experience proved inadequate, I did not go to look up the answer, but asked the master. And this frequently did happen, for as the reader will see there are things here that are too strange to accept without question.

But we should not be tempted to know better, to judge, or to assume that it is nonsense. Nothing is more damaging than prejudice. It is a thousand times worse than childish faith, which is also not desirable. In between lies a healthy skepticism which we can heartily recommend.

However, he who wants to read this book with profit, yet without starting to practice after the first few pages, should constantly try to bear in mind that there have been and still exist today human beings who through this peculiar practice reach a degree of self-control that is quite beyond our imagination.

Some will now say that I seem to think that I am the first one ever to speak about yoga, while they have known for some time how to evaluate the discipline. This may or may not be so. But I would ask the reader to start from scratch, as though he were an innocent child. Accept what is being said as something completely new, which in most respects it actually is: a translation of the most authoritative hatha yoga textbook of all times.

I imagine that I know a little about yoga, but when I stand before a master in India I become very quiet and humble. Forgetting that I know a little, I listen and learn. So far, this method has proved to be the most fruitful. There is time for philological studies when I am back in my room, where I can reflect upon what I have seen and heard.

Thus, in a sense, whoever takes up this book stands before a

13

very great master. May he be silent and listen, try to understand, and go to his earlier learning later to compare.

Here a new problem arises: the quest for a guru, which has now almost become a fad. And simultaneously another question, essential for Western students: Can a book replace the guru, the master? Not completely, of course. Still, the right book, read and understood correctly, can be more successful than running after a yoga master in India without understanding him, not realizing in our enthusiasm that he is not our guru; that he is a teacher, but not a guru. Not every teacher is a guru, and, strangely enough, not every guru is a teacher. He who uncritically trusts the first best yoga teacher—and they are as plentiful as sand at the seashore—may find that he has wasted his time and efforts with a gym teacher who knows no more (or even less) about the real goal of yoga than do his students. Unfortunately, this type of teacher is the most loquacious and most prolific. That is why most modern yoga books are superficial despite the beautiful Indian names of their authors. Most of these yogis did not go beyond the first two chapters of our text, and thus have not reached anything really decisive. The real yoga only begins where such yogis (and their books) end. No one has as yet reached any stage of enlightenment through physical exercises.

But we should talk about real gurus. Every human being yearns for the fulfillment of his most secret desires. Some, in order to be happy, seek nothing further than to learn the ABCs, while others will be happy with no less than the wisdom of God. Naturally, for the former the search for a teacher is simple. There are so many levels of desire between these two, in fact, that there are simply not enough kinds of gurus to meet the demand.

In reality things are a bit different, however. Our main problem at first is not to find *the* guru to lead the ignorant student on a spiritual apron-string to nirvana; rather is it important to progress by our own endeavor to the threshold of the closed door to final achievement, where only the experience and advice of a master can guide our ever more decisive and ever more dangerous steps. In other words, only when we have completely exhausted our own resources does the guru guide us to the solution of the last question, the final goal.

To prepare ourselves for a guru means self-discipline. In this sense, every sentence, even from the simplest book, has power to teach, if it happens (in a kind of negative polarity) to hit the corresponding vacuum in the reader's mind, and there fill a breach. Thus it can happen that we work our way through whole libraries and then find the key sentence in a newspaper. This sentence need not necessarily be very wise, but it must completely answer my question, mine and no one else's, for I am the one who is asking and the answer must give me some degree of enlightenment.

Those who expect an open door that they can enter without knocking may learn a great deal, but they will never reach the decisive knowledge. Only he who has learned long and with sacrifice can become a master. I know of no master who did not have to go through painful years of discipline. That these years were painful was not due to this so often accused "cruel world" and "hard life." Life is never hard if I am not too soft, if I am not afraid. The sage learns to be hard and unyielding toward himself. And behold, the world changes its face. Of course there is no universal recipe; every individual has his own weaknesses. But that things depend on the weakest part of our so complicated psyche-soul-body organism is undisputable, and we have to draw some conclusions from this fact. Let us take the greatest and perhaps most suffering seeker in world literature, Faust. . . . "Now here I stand, a simple fool, and am no wiser than before." He confesses that knowledge is not reached by being "smart" (worldly-wise). He knows his real aim without knowing how to reach it. He subscribes to the most impossible of all "sciences," to magic, in order to find out what ultimate force holds the world together. . . . Only he who goes beyond all words can reach the experience of reality.

It is not for the sake of mystery mongering that the highest teachings are as secret now as they have ever been. Were they to be given out indiscriminately to the novice who has no power of discrimination the guru would soon get a reputation as a devil who lightly hands out death and destruction. Secrecy is nothing but a protection for the student.

What does the guru really do? One readily imagines the student sitting day and night at the feet of the guru, being showered with secret teachings as a reward for having so diligently hunted for the guru. This would be nice, but completely useless.

What actually does happen? Let us take a seeker who does not yet quite know what in the deepest sense is at stake, nor has he any idea how to shape his spiritual future. He does not know which of the many yoga systems is right for him, but he is ready to strive and to submit himself to the wisdom of the master. And thus he goes in search of a guru.

Were it now as we would like to imagine, then by chance he would fall into the hands of a yoga teacher. Though chance has no place in yoga, it *is* left to chance whether he meets a yogi who can teach him mechanical technique or meets him whom he urgently needs. With bad luck he will run into any one of the above yogis, submit to him as a student and try to learn, only to find out after months or years that all remained empty and useless. Certainly he will have profited in some ways. But he will not feel that he has reached a higher stage of yoga. The teacher will not divulge to him the last secrets because he knows that this student is lacking the necessary foundation.

Usually, however, it happens that the student "accidentally" hears that somewhere there is a great saint. His teacher confirms this rumor. The student gets restless; perhaps his lack of success is the fault of the teacher. He wants to leave. His teacher has no objection, so he goes. The saint does not deign even to look at him. Impressed by the deep veneration shown to the master everywhere, he decides not to give up until the master accepts him as a student. Still the saint does not even look at the yearning one, says not a word. At most he waves him away once in a while. It is not pleasant to be so disliked and still remain. Thus days and weeks pass. He travels around with his haughty idol, or rather pursues him unremittingly for miles and miles. The only progress: the saint no longer waves him away. But still he does not look at him, nor does he speak to him. Until one day the miracle happens: the master looks at him and speaks one sentence; then he turns away, and the happy seeker no longer exists for him. That seeker can now quietly go home, for it is quite certain that he will not elicit another word from the guru.

What has happened here? Why does it seem so strange? First of all, let us discard the notion that the master did not heed the importunate student. Nothing during these weeks was to him more important than the student who did not notice the master's concern. Surely he tested the student; but more than this, he was master enough to know from his vibrations all the virtues and all the faults of that student. And when he finally decided to speak, it was only after he had formed his opinion. The opinion of a Western psychotherapist after years of depth analysis could not approach this master's in its absolute and complete certainty.

And the sentence? It contains—mostly in the form of a categorical imperative—the decisive wisdom which is to be the student's absolute leitmotiv for a number of years. Out of this sentence evolves everything that he now needs to accomplish his high goal. If he lives, thinks, and acts strictly according to the injunction of that sentence and continues with his previous yoga practice, he will suddenly see everything with new eyes, and the success he has been yearning for will materialize.

When we look at some of these sentences we are likely to be a little shocked by their apparent meaningless simplicity and exclaim: "What? Such a great saint has nothing more profound to say?" But we should not forget that psychotherapeutic prescriptions are the aim, not spirited phrases. The effectiveness of a medicine does not depend on its color or taste. What is essential is that it contain that which cures the body. The effect is what counts. The Amar Swami, a South Indian, a Pacceke Buddha, to my guru: "Take your reason and look." The Yoga Swami, a South Indian siddha: "Whatever happens has its meaning." And to the same student seven years later: "*Summa iru,*" which means both "be still" and "let go." Yogi Chellapa, also South Indian: "Make it new." These are just a few examples. One must not forget, however, that in the native language these sentences have a much deeper and more manifold meaning, and that through association their content is considerably enhanced. To submit such a sentence to psychological analysis would make sense only if we had a thorough acquaintance with the student involved.

In an easy and simple sentence we can test the effectiveness of such an approach. For one week ask yourself after everything you have done: "Was this necessary?" Was it necessary to be rude, to be angry? Was it necessary to let yourself go? Here is no hidden teaching, no yoga wisdom as one would like to have it presented. What it really means becomes evident only after one has carried the sentence around for a few weeks, having used it like a pair of spectacles through which to view everyday life. This is the answer to the riddle. The teaching of such a sentence does not necessarily make us "better." But we should become conscious of things we were previously hiding through fear, prudery, or negligence.

The guru knows intuitively what we most urgently need. But then he does not tell us directly. He lets us find out for ourselves, for only then are we really convinced. Open censure makes even the most devoted student rebellious. No matter how profound may be the teachings of a Buddha, a Christ, a Lao-tzu, a Mohammed, only what we discover for ourselves can immutably persuade us. This is the reason why we need a guru for these teachings that are often presented to us so clearly that we understand them intellectually, and why the guru then does not give us the decisive information, but indicates the ways and means to real knowledge. No book can proceed in such a manner. But once we have found them we also know which of the yoga systems is the most beneficial for us.

My guru in kundalini yoga is also a man of great learning in the shastras. One day I asked him for the meaning of certain symbols which seemed to me of great importance. "I cannot tell you this because you are not yet initiated." So I had to be patient.

When the time came, immediately after initiation I again asked the same question. "Meditate as I have told you before. Then you will experience." I was terribly disappointed, but had no choice but to obey. The result was that in a surprisingly short time I received the answer to my question, an answer that nobody could have given me in words. The symbolism in question was of such a deep nature that it could be grasped only by direct experience. The meditation that gave me the answer did not relay any intellectual association or hint; it only triggered off the process of understanding. This is the method of a real guru.

When the first guru has fulfilled his psychological aim and his "magic formula" has achieved its effect, the next guru, the yoga master (who is usually more accessible), begins to act, and we consult certain books, which undoubtedly can also help teach us. Key examples are the Upanishads, the Brahmanas, and the Tantras.

But here too it is not quite so simple. Not everything has equal value for everybody who hears. For example, a person wants to learn how to drive, so he buys a book that explains in detail how the motor works, and nobody tells him that this kind of knowledge alone will not make him a driver. When he has smashed up the car he realizes his lack of essential knowledge about driving. Actually, this is not a very good example, for the law puts the teacher before the license. But in yoga the law is still unwritten (though no less important), and that is why many a student has foundered.

As we will see from our text, what the West understands as yoga is simply a technique to keep the motor in good condition. This is eminently important, but is is not an end in itself. Our text claims—and rightly so—to be a yoga system (hatha yoga) that leads from what seems to be sheerly physical culture to the highest goal, raja yoga. The practice of the system presents comparatively few dangers for the student who does not overdo. No doubt danger exists, but I am sure that no reader will take an interest in those practices that are potentially dangerous. Fortunately, these are not particularly enticing, while the other, more attractive exercises are sufficient and rich enough to more than fill a lifetime of troubled city life.

So let us begin to read *Hatha Yoga Pradipika* by Yoga Swami Svatmarama. Put aside all your Western knowledge and your prejudice, and do what yoga students have done from time immemorial: sit down, relax, and listen with joyful attention to these ancient teachings. There will be ample time later on to accept or reject them.

PART ONE

THE FUNDAMENTAL PRINCIPLES

CHAPTER 1

THE PREREQUISITES

(1) Reverence to Siva the Lord of Yoga, who taught [his wife] Parvati hatha wisdom as the first step to the pinnacle of raja yoga.

It is a good practice to evoke a divine power before beginning serious work. We may call it Siva (the Benevolent) or God or Ganesa (*gana* = legions; *isa* = master), to whom in fact the yogi author has dedicated his work.

(2) Having thus solemnly saluted his master, Yogi Svatmarama now presents hatha vidya [vidya = wisdom] solely and exclusively for the attainment of raja yoga.

Now it can begin—and it begins with an admonition. The classical commentary, at times so tediously wordy, here has an important message: "solely for the attainment of raja yoga" indicates two delimitations. The lower level indicates that hatha yoga is not being taught for its own sake, for the achievement of physical fitness and worldly power, but is a method to prepare the student for the rigors of raja yoga.

The upper delimitation needs a little more elucidation. As we will soon and often hear, the real goal of a yogi is to become a siddha. A siddha, a person in possession of siddhis, has developed powers that can readily be called supernatural. There are eight siddhis, the highest of which is nirvana, the great liberation.

If in India, even with great masters, one so seldom has a chance to witness the miracles that these siddhas have the powers to perform, it is simply because a siddha who does not want to get the reputation of a black magician will keep his powers carefully concealed and refuse to use them for worldly purposes. If he does misuse a siddhi, the misused siddhi strikes back at him and causes him some kind of unpleasantness, usually of a physical nature.

One does not necessarily have to believe such things. You may put this down to the fabulous imagination of the East, and say so. The yogi does not resent your doubts, and they will not in any way impede the objective study of the wisdom of yoga. In fact, the text gives warning against striving primarily for powers: "solely for the attainment of raja yoga."

The deeper purpose of the siddhis is something else. Through the developing forces the student recognizes what stage of evolution he has reached. Certain phenomena will tell him that he should change his way of practice, and if after due practice these phenomena do not occur, he surely has made a mistake. The siddhis are signposts on his way to the final goal, liberation. To be a siddha means to be in possession of all the characteristics of the final yoga goal.

"Siddhis," my guru told me, "are not the aim of our work. We want to become siddhas in order to enjoy the realization and perfection of a siddha, not to gain worldly position or evade responsibilities." And since he himself is a siddha, this sentence clearly indicates what is defined as the upper delimitation. Yoga is not for braggarts or egocentrics, nor is it for those who merely want to add method to their physical training.

(3) For those who wander in the darkness of conflicting creeds [and philosophies], unable to reach to the heights of raja yoga

24

[*self-knowledge and cosmic consciousness*] *the merciful Yogi Svatmarama has lit the torch of hatha wisdom.*

Raja yoga, the royal yoga,[1] is a goal that many strive to reach without even being aware of it, without having the slightest inkling of yoga. What else is Faust aspiring to but perfect self-knowledge and cosmic consciousness, to "know that force which holds the universe together, to see creative power and the seed"?

For the student of Indian wisdom this reference to Faust presents an especially interesting parallel. Goethe speaks here of creative power and of seed, in Sanskrit *shakti* and *bindu*, two of the most important terms in tantra yoga, as we will see later on. At the time of Goethe these teachings had not yet reached the West, and it speaks for his universal genius that he recognized their supreme importance.

(4–9) *Goraksha and Matsyendra were masters of hatha vidya, and by their grace Yogi Svatmarama learned it. Siva, Matsyendra, Shabara, Anandabhairava, Chaurangi, and many other great siddhas who have conquered time are still roaming through this world.*

A daring statement: after the enumeration of 33 masters of hatha vidya who have illuminated the ages, to claim that they are still roaming through the world, for "they have conquered time."

We have already spoken of the siddhis, and here it is specifically stated that these masters were siddhas. They reached what so many covet, "eternal youth." Many are the tales of yogis who are said to be several hundred years old and look like youths, but it is useless to discuss this kind of doubtful rumor. A wandering

1. The translation of the term "raja yoga" as "royal yoga" is exoteric. Esoterically it is "the yoga of radiating light," for "*raja*" can also mean "to shine." Thus we have an allusion to the "inner light," which is dealt with in the fourth part of this work.

yogi has no birth certificate, and it seems strange that one can state that he is exactly 250 years old, while his younger colleagues do not know whether they are 15, 20, 30, or 40 years old. Besides, a hundred years more or less is important only to us. To a yogi who lives alone in the woods time is of no concern. True, I did meet some yoga masters who looked younger than their grown sons, and this alone seems quite a desirable goal. And it is also true what is stated above: that these yoga masters had conquered time. That is, they were no longer subject to the laws of time; they were masters of this strange unfathomable mystery, "time."

For us time is inseparable from the clock, but no one has ever succeeded in really defining time. It is impossible—because time does not exist outside of our own minds. As our consciousness, so our time: long as eternity the hour of danger; short and fleeting the hour of happiness. So when we say that a yogi has conquered time it means that he has conquered his (relative) consciousness.

(10) [Therefore] hatha yoga is a refuge for all those who are scorched by the three fires. To those who practice yoga, hatha yoga is like the tortoise that supports the world.

These three fires are well known to us; they are the fire of self-created suffering; the fire of suffering through higher powers; and the fire of suffering that is caused by other beings.

Nobody can eliminate from this world the influences that create such sufferings. What we can and should do is to prepare the physical-mental-spiritual soil in such a way that the seed of impressions cannot sprout into suffering.

Sufferings are unfulfilled desires. The realization of these desires depends not only on ourselves, but is subject primarily to external influences. If I want something, I have to try to reach it.

For this I am dependent on my own power as against the opposing forces. And we always desire something, even if it is the desire for the happiness of a desireless state.

Now we are on the track of our idea: to be desirelessly happy means to want nothing, to have no needs, to be happy with oneself and the given conditions. But yoga does not mean to learn self-satisfaction. Rather, it means to strive for such a state of perfection that some day it will be our nature to be desirelessly happy—and to have good reason for it.

This is by no means a state of apathy, devoid of the dynamics of natural activities. On the contrary, our endeavors will no longer be whipped by passions toward a goal where, with open eyes, we uselessly invest our most precious forces in senseless intoxication. We will learn to evaluate our wishes, to know our own forces as well as the opposing powers. And if we have to renounce, we will then do so with clear understanding, not with a painful sensation of loss.

As to the symbolism of the tortoise, this is a meaningful legend which we will encounter later and which will accompany us throughout the whole book.

(11) A yogi who is desirous of developing siddhis should keep the hatha yoga strictly secret, for only then will he have success. All his efforts will be in vain if he reveals everything without discrimination.

Physical exercises are nothing shameful, and they are fun; but practiced on a highway they become insanity. "When you pray, go into a room by yourself." Or, more drastically: "Do not cast pearls before swine."

(12) The student of hatha yoga should practice in a solitary place, in a temple or a hermitage, an arrow shot away from rocks, water, and fire. The land should be fertile and well governed.

27

Here we have the first great problem, larger perhaps than that of the siddhis: to find a quiet spot, undisturbed and safe. Predatory animals, earthquakes, and floods: those were the problems at that time. Today's problems are professional, financial, political, which constantly drag the practitioner back into the stream of social life.

However, it is not entirely impossible to create a hermitage under modern conditions. Perhaps there is a quiet attic, away from the attractions of movies, radio, television, where we can meet our neglected and ignored own selves.

(13) The hermitage should have a small door and no windows. It should be level with the ground and have no holes in the wall. [It should be] neither too high nor too long, and clean and free from insects. It should be laid daily with cow dung. Outside there should be a raised platform with an elevated seat and a water tank. The whole should be surrounded by a wall. These are the characteristics of a yoga hermitage as described by the siddhas, the masters of hatha yoga.

Do not despair! I have seen many hemitages that conformed in only a few points to the ideal. Some had holes in the walls and most of them were lacking the cow dung. But all of them were clean. We should not be too dependent on external conditions, helpful though they may be. If I so *will*, my hermitage has neither doors or windows. And when I am distracted, my restless mind will penetrate the thickest walls. If the hermitage is not ideal, a little extra effort must be made. The goal of yoga is by no means dependent on cow dung.

(14) Seated in such a place, the yogi should free his mind from all distracting thoughts and practice yoga as instructed by his guru.

28

Our keenest weapon, and often our only salvation, is our thought power. If your thought is open, so is the chance of success; if it is slow and limited, you will be left behind in the great race for success. Not only is *right* thought essential, but also the capacity to think of several things simultaneously. Many Western men with executive ulcers could write reams about this.

Must men be like this? Evidently, if they wish to succeed. But what is success? Nothing against success—which, after all, is the foundation of a "happy life." Success is wealth, wealth is happiness; therefore, success is happiness. A logical conclusion, but somehow it leaves us uneasy. Is the man who has bought success with his health, with the sacrifice of his most precious attribute, really happy?

There is a different way. One of the most remarkable men of our time, and by no means a pious man, swears by yoga. Every morning Pandit Nehru, the coolest thinker of his country and a maker of world history, stood on his head, and with him 63 members of Congress. Yehudi Menuhin, the great violinist, makes no secret about his yoga. And like him many of the most successful men of our day, including medical men who are world famous, find in yoga the purest source of human harmony.

Harmony: the key word, the all-important. There is no objection to the search for success as long as the harmony of life is not disturbed. No need to relinquish any of our plans and principles as long as there is harmony.

How does harmony come about? The very question proves that this fundamental law of life is becoming more and more a myth as we are turned more and more into machines. So let us try to find the yoga way to harmony.

(15) The yoga forces are dissipated by too much eating, heavy physical labor, too much talk, the observances of [ascetic] vows, [promiscuous] company, and a growling stomach [too much fasting].

Here we have the disharmonies of everyday life, and not even the great ones. Not distrust, not rudeness, not lack of consideration, not anger and despair. Just immoderation. And that is bad enough.

The yogi never quite fills his stomach; the executive always does. The yogi is healthy; the executive has ailments. Harmony versus disharmony.

(16) Success depends on a cheerful disposition, perseverance, courage, self-knowledge, unshakable faith in the word of the guru, and the avoidance of all [superfluous] company.

Again the magic word of our time: success. And with it even a formula. Nothing about overtime, or night work, and "you must . . ." Not even a word about thinking.

A cheerful disposition is incompatible with executive ulcers. Perseverance! That sounds promising. But the keynote is harmony, and the perseverance referred to here is not that of the executive's marathon conference.

But don't forget that yoga has not yet begun. We are stating here only the minimal prerequisites without which any attempt at practice would be senseless. These preliminary requirements can be fulfilled by anyone, and they will bestow more happiness upon you than you would expect—without exercise, without risk. (Once we really embark upon yoga, however, the evasion of a single requirement can turn nectar into poison.)

Yoga practice, regardless of the system we follow, has a psychological depth effect. One exercise goes in this direction, another in that. Often they have a perplexing similarity; here and there we find a minimal difference which seems inconsequential. The guru, however, watches not so much the exercises in general, but just those little details. The student does not know why and is liable to ridicule such pettiness; but the guru knows our needs better than we do. He knows that each physical action has its psychic-spiritual reflex, just as every psychic-spiritual attitude is manifest in the body.

Western science too is aware of the inseparable interrelation between body, soul, and mind. A bit of iodine, adrenaline, or cortisone will change our whole world view. Our whole life is chemically conditioned. Every thought activates one or the other nerve center which in turn influences some endocrine gland. The gland sends its hormones into the bloodstream, we react, new thoughts arise which in turn again influence a nerve center and create new reactions, combining with other nerve centers. There are many centers, many glands, and countless combinations. And this cycle is only one of the inner processes affected by yoga.

If a certain practice hits something unhealthy (an asana can touch on an organic illness, a deep meditation on some mental suffering), then the result is not as desired; it can even lead to disaster. Quite often nature helps itself. But in very deep meditation (which is hardly ever allowed without initiation) some very powerful phenomena can appear which will frighten the weak into refraining from further investigation. That is why the passage above calls for courage.

One thing is certain: these preliminary chapters are the most important part of the book. He who disregards them should certainly consider yoga dangerous.

(17a) Not to cause suffering to any living being; to speak the truth; not to take what belongs to others; to practice continence; to develop compassion and fortitude; to be merciful to all and honest; to be moderate in eating and pure in heart. These are the first prerequisites of yoga [the yamas]. Self-limitation [tapas, austerities], *cheerfulness, religious faith, charity, contemplation, listening to sacred scriptures, modesty, a clean mind, recitation of*

mantras [japa], and observance of rules, these are the second re-quirements of yoga [the niyamas].

Thus equipped one can venture to take the first step into the wonderland of one's own self. You do not have to take all the rules literally, but you have to look at them seriously. Not the word "yoga," but the power behind it, is decisive. And this power? *"Tat tvam asi!*—Thou art That!"

CHAPTER 2

YOGA AND THE ART OF HEALING

IN Japan there are physicians who kick the patient in the back, twist his neck, or simply give him a heavy slap on the shoulder, and the patient feels like a new man. In China there are physicians who practice acupuncture (the insertion of needles). They prick a place quite apart from the ailing organ and pain disappears—quite suddenly. In Ceylon there are doctors who touch the patient's skin with a red hot iron—and they aim with the precision of a fraction of a millimeter. A quick pain. The patient is cured.

These are not medicine men at work. Here we have full-fledged physicians who master an art—that nobody in the West can understand? These times have passed. The example of the Japanese doctors has proven itself a hundred times. In America chiropractice has become an academic discipline.

Thus too it is with acupuncture. We now have theses on the subject, as well as practicing Western physicians. The third example (Ceylon) too will no doubt some day be accepted, perhaps along with some practices of medicine men that we ridiculed some 50 years ago. Primitive people are really not as primitive as we in our arrogant prejudice are apt to imagine. Are not the methods of modern politicians more primitive than those of a medicine man in the jungle?

We want to study the following chapters on asanas and their psycho-physical background with this in mind.

"Why so many words?" some will ask. "Asanas are physical exercises." And in a sense he is right.

"Nonsense," another will say, "all these senseless contortions." And in a sense he too is right.

A third will consider asanas a practice that nobody can quite understand. Right too.

A fourth one stands thoughtfully in a corner. "I will learn to understand the inner connections. I have studied medicine and will soon find out what bodily functions are involved. I cannot imagine that the yogis have taken all this out of thin air. There must be a corresponding scientific terminology." Beware of this man.

Each of the first three critics acknowledged a certain positive aspect of the practice. The first speaks of gymnastics and expects no more than the success of gymnastics. Very good. One should approach these practices not with vague expectations but with clear purposefulness. After all, only the literature of the West presents these preliminary exercises with such great mystification, whereas in comparison with what follows after them they are really little more than gymnastics.

Nor should he who speaks of meaningless contortions be condemned. Perhaps he is right. For who is capable of explaining the internal relationships? Why give the contortions a meaning for which we have not the slightest proof—except for a few books whose value the average Western reader is unable to ascertain? This skeptic is not likely to start practice, but he is justified in his statement if by "sense" he understands that which can be clearly defined by our intellect. These are practices that "nobody can really understand" because they reach too deeply into our inner world, touch on areas that have not yet been named. From this angle no sense can be discovered, just as it cannot be convincingly denied. It is only the Westerner who seeks "sense" in everything. The Asiatic accepts mystery as a fact, and thus the "senseless," in an intellectual sense, becomes for him sense (in relation to his experience). He experiences the *value* of that which we cannot understand.

The fourth is the dangerous one, for he swears by his intellectual knowledge alone. He has studied, he is perfect, he cannot err. (And imagine him as a student of a medicine man.) Science has canonized our intellect, and acknowledges nothing as superior, or even equal to it. Fortunately, we have the really great like C. G. Jung, Erwin Rousselle, and others who have gone to the "primitive" to expand their knowledge.

Nobody will claim that our knowledge acquired through the centuries is wrong. No, it is completely right, but utterly incomplete because it is so one-sided. There are more things in heaven and earth than are dreamt of in academia, things that we know exist and that we cannot fathom with our scientifically trained intellect.

"Well," he will say if he is judicious, "I admit this, but we must have a certain frame of reference. It is quite clear that chakras are nerve centers and nadis represent nerve strands. Why should we deny this? Knowing this does make it easier." However convincing these words may sound, they contain the seed of the greatest error in yoga: foundering through thought. In other words, the dangerous supposition that the essential can be fathomed by thought, that it is "nothing but," that with a little effort of our conceptual intellect we can descend to the very depths of our soul, to the foundation of the universe. Certainly this trend of thought is logical, but what good is logic when yoga wisdom is beyond logic?

This phrase has discredited yoga with the intellectuals. But let us look at our lives. Is life always logical? Where is the logic of the scientist who analyzes natural laws six days a week and on the seventh goes to church to pray to a God who has no place in his logical system of science? Where is the logic of the drug addict who knows he is digging his grave and still does not desist? Where is the logic of the greedy old man who, with one foot in the grave still craves millions, though he cannot take a penny with him? Is the cosmic mathematics of Einstein which created our atomic age limited to logic? And how about the fate of the evil rich man and the virtuous poor? Is chance logical? No, the decisive factors of our existence have nothing to do with logic, and therefore we can readily postulate that the essential interrelations in yoga cannot be penetrated by logical deductions, which, however, does not mean that there is no law.

When we seem to detect an analogy between a certain concept in yoga and a Western scientific term we must at once deny ourselves all further investigations of an analogy. Why? When one mistakes the part for the whole, as often happens in Western science, one underestimates the whole because one applies to it the lesser value of the part. And how can we possibly judge anything if we know only one of its many facets, and not even the most essential one at that? Take the example of the chakras, the centers of power, which are often identified with chief nerve centers (ganglia), or with main glands, simply because there is a topographical similarity. With this we confuse cause and effect.

Although we know very little about the central nervous system and the glands, we do know enough to gauge their effects. But what we can learn about chakras in yoga is immense. If the system of chakras were identical with the central nervous system (CNS), then either all our academic knowledge would be wrong, or the yoga teachings would be empty fantasies. But neither is the case. Our knowledge about the CNS applies to the material aspect only, while chakra theory goes to the deepest sources of all dynamic processes in man, down to the deepest cosmic functions, to which we are undeniably bound. There are many effects resulting from the activity of the CNS and the glands which will forever remain a mystery if we ignore the much subtler aspects of these chakras.

It is characteristic that the tantric Buddhism of Tibet teaches that the yogi has to *create* the chakras at the relevant places in his body. They are so to speak "psychic centers" that cannot be practically recognized unless I will it. They are vibration centers which are developed in the course of yoga practice. This alone proves how elusive they are to the surgeon's knife.

But we have not yet come to these strange things. First now to the "gymnastics" of hatha yoga. Even here we should deny ourselves any profound speculations. Certainly one could—and even with a fair measure of success—draw psychosomatic conclusions from asana such-and-such. But again, logic deserts us after a certain point and what remains cannot be investigated by science, however fine its intentions. And this would mean: beyond the borderline of logic there "really" is nothing. But actually a great deal is there; not only is it there now, but it has been there since the very beginning. The logician does not have to bother about all this, of course, since he has a wealth of concrete, factual material at his disposal.[2]

In any event, whether or not certain pranayamas (breathing exercises) regulate the oxygen content of our blood is none of our concern. What is important for us is that forces (currents) are being activated that no Western scientist is able fully to evaluate, but which are the very foundation of the whole yoga structure.

Therefore, Western science, despite its undisputed merits, will be neglected in the following chapters, in favor of that ancient science which is the foundation of yoga therapy. This, I think, is much more vital for the understanding of "Eastern exotics." We should try to think Indian while studying this book—Indian not

2. "At the borderline of logic science stops, but not nature, which blossoms there where no theory has as yet penetrated" (C. G. Jung, *The Psychology of Transference*).

only in relation to yoga, but also in relation to the presuppositions of yoga.

The art of healing, like all else truly Indian, is based on the Vedas, the oldest book of humanity. Everything that concerns medical theory in the Rig-Veda, the Sama-Veda, the Atharva-Veda, and the Yajur-Veda, was later systematized into Ayurvedic medicine.

Although it is not possible to summarize this gigantic work, which is still in practical use in India today, much less give a survey of the wealth of its principles, we can at least consider the three main concepts of human physiology upon which this system is based. This is important because prejudiced Westerners who cast a superficial eye upon the standard work of Ayurvedic medicine, the *Charaka Samhita*, have misinterpreted thoroughly these three concepts.

The teaching states that there are three dominant forces in man, and accordingly three main sources of illness: vata, pitta, and kapha. The usual translations as wind, gall, and phlegm are misleading, incomplete, senseless, and simply wrong—as wrong as the false analogies discussed earlier. All three terms are infinitely more complex and become meaningful only in their completeness. To understand the terms vata, pitta, and kapha we need the help of the classical definitions. Comprehension of these terms is all the more important because hatha yoga is closely bound to ayurvedic principles, as we soon shall see.

The three terms encompass all physiological functions of the human body, and their imbalance causes not only illness but also susceptibility to contagious diseases.

Vata

It is true that this word means "wind" literally. But more important is the root *va,* movement. To quote the *Charaka Sam-*

hita: "Vata is the source of both structure and function [of the body]. It is that which is represented by the five forms [of the bodily currents]: prana, udana, samana, vyana, and apana. It is the initiator of the upward and downward flow [of all internal processes such as circulation, metabolism, etc.]; the controller and guiding force of consciousness; the stimulant of the senses; the companion of sensations; the organizer of the elements of the body; the principle of synthesis; the storage battery of speech; the cause of feelings and perception; the origin of excitement and stimulation; it fans the gastric fire, dries out harmful phlegm; expels excrements; is purifier of the coarse and the fine channels of the body; the creator of the fetal form; the principle of life preservation. All these are the normal functions of vata in our body" (*Char. Sam.* I. 12:8). Disturbance of any one of these functions leads to illness and susceptibility to infection.

Some of the illnesses due to the influence of vata are: rheumatism, dislocations, lameness, cramps, stiffness of limbs, peristaltic irregularities, trembling, emotional and depressive states, everything related to tension, relaxation, expansion and contraction, circulation and metabolism, crookedness and distortion of limbs, abdominal diseases, menstrual irregularities, sterility, hallucinations, and convulsions.

Pitta

This can be translated as "gall," but here it implies rather that which is also expressed by the word gall: temperament. But this again only in a limited sense. The *Charaka Samhita* derives this word from the root *tap,* "to heat," and this brings us closer to the meaning. We quote: "It is only the fire which in pitta brings on good and bad results, according to the normal or abnormal condition [of the organs]. The results are digestion and indigestion, power of perception and its loss, normal and abnormal body temperatures, healthy and unhealthy look, temerity, fear [nerves], anger and joy [moods], confusion and clarity, and other such contrasting pairs" (*Char. Sam.* I. 12:11). "The normal function of pitta causes: power of cognition, fire of digestion, fresh complexion, clarity of thought, body temperature, hunger and thirst, and nimbleness of mind" (*Char. Sam.* I. 18:50). Diseases from this source are: inflammation, fever, pus, perspiration, softening of bodily substance, itching, metabolic irregularities, redness, bad odor and taste, as well as discoloration.

Kapha

This word is composed of two roots: *ka* = "water," and *pha*, which refers to the process of biological evolution. And since we know that the body is largely composed of liquid we could translate *kapha* as "life-fluid."

"Kapha is the nectar [soma]. It is the fertile water for the play of life; it is living fluid, the protoplasm that sustains all life processes; it is indeed the scaffold of life. It binds the limbs together and produces all the connecting, nourishing, developing, and fortifying functions. It promotes the well-being of the body by its lubricating action. Thus it supplies the water for the roots of life. In its physiological aspect [!] kapha is the power and perseverance of man, which, however, immediately becomes a disturbing impurity when his balance is disturbed" (*Char. Sam.* I. 12:12). Kapha ailments are: pallidness, cold, edema, constipation, diabetes, secretions, cold sweat, languidness, and swellings (tumors).

"No pain without vata (the stream of life), no inflammation without pitta (the fire of life), no swellings without kapha (the fluid of life)." This clearly shows the coordination of the three forces, but it also demonstrates—and more clearly than Western medicine does—the interdependence of body and mind.

40

Naturally the ancient Indian art of healing is not exhausted by these three main terms. On the contrary, this is only the beginning. For us, however, this short survey will suffice. It will elucidate much that is to follow; in fact, much would be unintelligible without it.

We must not forget that these three "doshas" have a material-bodily, as well as an ethereal and an abstract-spiritual aspect. Thus when later on we deal extensively with the prana, the life stream that here is "vata," then with "soma," the nectar, the "fertile water for the play of life" that here is "kapha," and finally with the inner fire that is "pitta," we should not forget this survey. Soon we will learn that all the wisdom of physiological healing also has its place in higher spiritual spheres.

For the Indian there is one straight path through the universe and situated on this path are all the cities of the world: medicine, philosophy, mathematics, astrology and astronomy, physics, logic, sports, magic, etc., and to him who is fully conversant with any one of them, the others are no secret.

So let us start by looking at yoga with a new physiological understanding. Not so much to relearn, but to understand that there is wisdom in things that seem quite odd to us.

CHAPTER 3

THE ASANAS

(17b) Asanas are spoken of first, being the first stage of hatha yoga. So one should practice the asanas, which give [the yogi] strength, keep him in good health, and make his limbs supple.

Our concern is not yet with raja yoga and its mysteries. Let us first concentrate on strength, health, and litheness of body. Much of this will be of direct help in raja yoga.

(18) I shall now proceed to impart some of the asanas that were adopted by such wise men as Vasishtha, and practiced by yogis like Matsyendra.

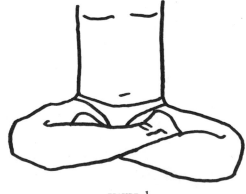

FIGURE 1

42

(19) Sitting straight on level ground, squeeze both feet between calves and thighs [of the opposite legs]. This is svastikasana. [See Figure 1.]

(20) Place the right foot under the left buttock and the left foot under the right buttock. This is gomukhasana, and looks like the mouth of a cow. [See Figure 2.]

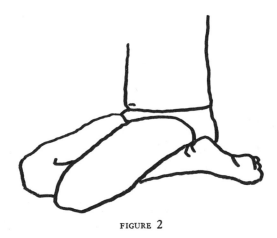

FIGURE 2

(21) Place one foot upon the other thigh and the other foot below the opposite thigh. This is virasana. [See Figure 3.]

In the last three phrases we simply have variations of sitting cross-legged as has been customary in India for thousands of years. These asanas in themselves are not practice; rather, they are fundamental conditions upon which the real practice is based. The following sentence is a continuation of the instructions of No. 20.

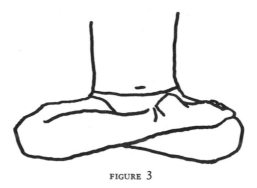

FIGURE 3

(22) Press the anus firmly with crossed feet and sit thus. But do it with care. This is ḳurmasana.

Here we might look for a deeper meaning, since the posture does not really bear any characteristics of gymnastics. We cannot yet understand the significance of the pressure on the anus, and the special emphasis on care. But at this point, of course, the student knows nothing yet about the essentials.

(23) Assuming the lotus posture, insert the hands between the thighs and calves. Put the hands firmly on the ground and raise the body up. This is ḳuḳḳutasana. [See Figure 4.]

The lotus posture has not yet been mentioned: the feet are placed crosswise on the opposite thighs, as close to the body as possible. Push the hands through this "network" of legs and place them firmly on the ground.

Here we have what clearly seems a gymnastic exercise. Yet what is involved is something quite different. Much later we will learn that to "raise the kundalini" a little help is needed, and this asana provides it. It may seem a difficult asana. But things get even more complicated in the following:

44

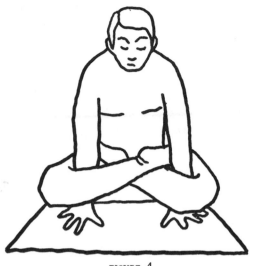

FIGURE 4

(24) Assuming the [above-mentioned] kukkutasana posture, put both arms around your neck and remain raised like a tortoise [with the back touching the ground]. This is uttana kurmasana.

Here the gymnastic character is evident; in fact it seems so exaggeratedly acrobatic that we wonder whether this is less than gymnastics—or more? What is behind it? *Kurma asana* means "tortoise posture." With a little imagination we can think of the body in this position as a tortoise. But strangely enough reference here is to something quite different.

So far we have encountered the tortoise three times. First in No. 10: "To those who practice yoga, hatha yoga is like the tortoise that carries the world." In the second place (No. 22) the asana in which the anus is pressed is called "tortoise posture" (kurmasana). And now here in No. 24 we have "the raised tortoise" (uttana kurmasana). Let us look at the ancient texts.

In the *Bhagavat Purana,* one of the richest of the ancient texts of Indian mythology and symbolism, we find a legend which is more than merely a legend. In a battle with the demons the gods were losing: they had considered themselves divinely superior to the forces of the world (the demoniac), but these forces stood more safely and firmly upon their ground. Brahma, whom the gods implored for help, ascended with the threatened ones to the Lord of the World, Vishnu, to ask his advice.

"Make peace with the demons," he urged them, "and churn with their help the nectar of immortality. The divine alone is as powerless as the earthly alone. Together you should churn the ocean of milk until it turns into the nectar of immortality."

So together the sworn enemies took the mountain Mandara, the backbone of the universe, wound around it the serpent Vasuki in three and one-half turns, and alternately pulling on the head (the demons) and the tail (the gods), they began to churn the terrestrial ocean of milk.

But soon the mountain became too heavy for the diligent ones, and slowly it sank lower and lower. Then Vishnu transformed himself into a tortoise, dove to the bottom of the ocean, and raised the mountain so that the work could be completed.

Practically every word in this legend is the expression of a deep symbolism, much of which will be clarified in the course of our study and practice. For now let us consider only the most important points. Not only in modern medicine, but in ancient yoga as well, the spinal column is the most important and most subtle part of the body. In fact we shall soon see that it is actually the spinal column that has the most important task.

Upon this "axis of the [human] universe" we exert pressure in kurmasana, so that the combined forces of the divine (subconscious) and the earthly (conscious) can accomplish their task. Most asanas involve the spinal column, as does the following:

(25) Grasp both toes with the hands [left with left, right with

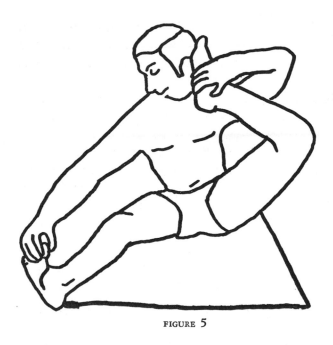

FIGURE 5

right], *keep one leg straight and draw the other to the ear as you would the string of a bow. This is dhanurasana. (See Figure 5.)*

The spinal cord has two ends: the earth (below) and heaven (above), as is fitting for a "holy mountain in the center of the world." And—as it should be—the worldly problems are mostly situated in the lower part and the more ideal ones in the upper one. We cannot be expected to comprehend this. That the earthly problems are centered in the lower half of the body only he who knows something about the chakras can realize. The yogi develops understanding only in the third stage.

We could compare ourselves with a tree that has its roots in the earth and the crown with its fruit in the sky. Just as we have to satisfy the needs of the roots in order to supply nourishment to the fruit in the crown, so most asanas are designed to cultivate the root of our tree of life, the spinal column.

As is this asana:

(26) Place your right foot on the outside of the left hip joint and the left foot outside the right knee [which is flat on the floor]. Grasp the left foot with the right hand [passing the arm to the left side of the knee] and the right one with the left hand. Turn the head all the way over to the left. This is matsyendrasana. [See Figure 6.]

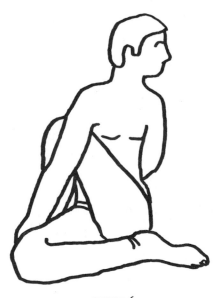

FIGURE 6

In the more current variations of this asana the right foot is not grasped by the left hand; instead, the hand is placed on the back as far over as possible. This is seen in our illustration.

Slight variations in asanas or occasional variations in name have

48

arisen because several teachers developed the same asanas. The variations occur only in minor points. This becomes quite evident by a comparison of our *Hatha Yoga Pradipika* with the more common and much later work, the *Gheranda Samhita*.

(27) This matsyendrasana increases the appetite by fanning the gastric fire [pitta], and destroys physical ailments. Kundalini is awakened and the moon made steady.

For the first time the text mentions kundalini, a latent force of highest potential, said to lie in three and one-half coils, like the snake in the churning of the ocean of milk, sleeping at the lowest center (muladhara chakra) at the foot of the "tree of life," the spinal column. This serpent power, kundalini, cannot be described fully, even by one who has succeeded in awakening it. When it awakens, it shoots through the body like an electric shock, and, trembling and amazed, the person realizes that a powerful event has taken place within him. This is only the beginning.

The whole body trembles. A door seems to have been pushed open through which a flood of light flows from some unknown world, a light of incomparable radiance. After a long time the trembling body becomes calm, but the flash of light shooting through the spinal column to the crown of the head is unforgettable.

This flash of light is not really the kundalini, however. It is merely a sign of its awakening. The kundalini itself does not shoot up, but will later rise slowly, passing through the stations (the chakras), each of which creates another new and powerful experience.

Whether the kundalini can really be awakened through this particular asana alone is questionable. But the asana will surely be helpful in the process. And the "moon"?

As mentioned above, the "mountain in the center of the world" has the earth at its foot and the sky at its peak. Between earth and sky are the sun (the center of the planetary system) and the moon.

In the center of the triangle formed by the navel and the two nipples is the "sun" [solar plexus]; at the upper end of the spinal column, at the medulla oblongata, sits the "moon." "Sun" and "moon" are not chakras but are spheres that stand directly under the influence of two chakras, lying respectively just above and below.

Through this asana the "moon" sphere is "massaged," which is all the more important as it is presumably here that we find the source of the fluid of life (kapha). But also the opposite pole, the "sun," is affected by this process of twisting the spinal column. And since it is here that the "fire of life" (pitta) originates, there arises from the combined work of these two well-springs a powerful stimulating influence upon the physiology of the body.

(28) Stretch out both legs and, taking hold of the toes, lay your head upon the knees. This is paccimasana [pashimottarasana].

(29) This most excellent of all asanas causes the breath to flow through the sushumna, fans the fire of appetite [pitta], *makes the loins supple* [vata] *and removes all ailments* [caused by pitta and vata].

The most essential phrase of this sloka needs elucidation. Sushumna is the name for the hair-thin channel that traverses the spinal column lengthwise. It is the pathway of kundalini. Is the breath really to flow through this channel? It seems physiologically impossible. "Breath" in Sanskrit is *prana*; but what we call breath is only an insignificent fraction of what the Indian understands by prana. Breath is more than inhaled and exhaled air, more than oxygen and nitrogen, even more than any chemist could analyze. Breath is the carrier of an especially efficacious life force, of a stream which nourishes the organism. There is actually little difference between this "life current" and an eleccal current.

Enough about prana for now. (There will be a great deal more about it in later chapters.) Here again in this asana we see what seems to be a purely physical exercise, but it is one with a very specific meaning and aim.

(30) Press your hands firmly upon the ground and balance your body by pressing the elbows against your loins. Raise your legs straight in the air till your feet are level with your head. This is mayurasana. [See Figure 7.]

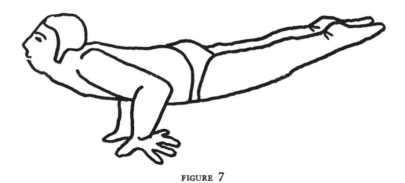

FIGURE 7

(31) This asana heals various diseases of the spleen and dropsy, and removes all illnesses caused by excess of vata, pitta, or kapha. It digests an overabundance of food, and even destroys the poison halahala.

The asana looks like our well-known gymnastic exercise on the parallel bars. And gymnastics it is. At this point of training the plan is to perfect the body and especially to train the abdominal muscles so important in Parts Two and Three of this work.

As the gods and the demons were diligently churning the ocean of milk and the ocean gradually began to change, the demons sampled the liquid and doubled over in great pain because the first product was sheer poison (halahala). In order to prevent further trouble, Siva swallowed the remaining poison. It remained in his throat and turned it blue.

At this stage of development the student does not understand the deeper meaning of the story, and does not yet know that it is a romantic allegory of his own development. He is glad to hear that Siva drank the poison, and believes that he is therefore out of danger, until he later learns that danger will still threaten if he does not carefully follow his guru's instructions. And he does not know that the poison is not a chemical but a spiritual poison, a psychic danger which arises from wrong practice.

Here again the question arises how this single asana can have such far-reaching consequences that it renders the poison harmless. In order to judge we must know two things: first, what kind of danger is referred to; second, what effects are produced by this asana.

We shall discuss this question to give the Western student a deeper insight, although it does not really belong here.

As mentioned before, the whole Indian mythology has a direct relation to yoga. When the universe (macrocosm) is mentioned, it is also a reference to man (microcosm). And under "gods and demons" we must understand the forces that are manifest in man on the psychic, mental, and physical levels.

Thus the churning of the ocean is, generally speaking, a process in yoga. This milk ocean symbolizes the brain. In the course of yoga training there occurs a transformation of consciousness from the "milk of devotional thinking" through the "poison of imperfect development" to the "nectar of enlightenment." In the state of incomplete evolution lies the greatest danger, i.e., premature action resulting from erroneous, ill-informed judgment. The student assumes he possesses certain powers, and may even have seen some indication of these, but he is not yet capable of recognizing and governing them. And this is poison, especially for further development. It is now imperative to mobilize counterforces.

In mayurasana the pressure of both elbows seals off the "prana channels" of the two nadis and thus forces an increased blood supply into those parts of the brain that are in most urgent need of it.

It seems clear that the blood suffusion of the brain must have an influence on our consciousness, but blood itself is less important than the stream of prana which imparts itself to the bloodstream. It is, so to speak, an electrification of the brain, a change of gear in the psychic mechanism. And it has been proven a thousand times that a clear head is the result of yoga practice.

(32) Lying full length on the back like a corpse is called savasana. With this asana tiredness caused by other asanas is eliminated; it also promotes calmness of mind.

How nice that relaxation is part of the scheme. And it is pleasant to find that no mystery is involved. Simply stretch out on the floor.

But this relaxation is also necessary, as that which follows is more thorough, has greater depth. We are about to take an important step in the direction of raja yoga.

(33–34) The asanas taught by Siva are 84 in number. Of these I will describe four of the most important ones. They are siddhasana, padmasana, simhasana, and bhadrasana. Of these, siddhasana is the best and most comfortable posture.

53

(35) Press one heel into the place below the sex organs [the perineum] *and put the other heel just above this region* [*close to the abdomen*]. *Press the chin upon the chest, sit up straight, with controlled organs, and fasten the eyes between the eyebrows. This is siddhasana, whereby all obstacles on the path to perfection are removed.* [*See Figure 8.*]

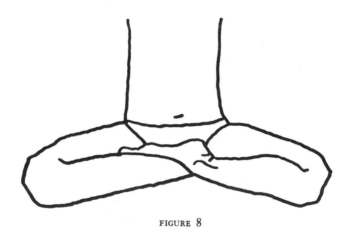

FIGURE 8

It is quite clear that more is at play here than mere gymnastic exercise, especially since there is no longer any mention of healing or nimble limbs.

But what do these unusual details mean? Each heel presses a certain point, the lower one the muladhara chakra, the upper one the svadhistana chakra. The neck is bent so as to press the vishuddha chakra in the throat, and the eyes are turned toward the ajna chakra.

The manipura chakra in the diaphragm region and the anahata chakra in the heart region seem to remain unnoticed. In reality it is just the contrary. The heart chakra has a unique position in many ways; it would not respond to physical pressure in any event. In this position it can be influenced by a meditative process, as we will see later on.

The manipura chakra is also dealt with in an unusual manner here, for instructions are static in nature. A later sloka (41) will add a dynamic element that will affect the manipura chakra, among other things.

(36) Place the right heel above the sex organ and the left heel over the right. This too is siddhasana. [See Figure 9.]

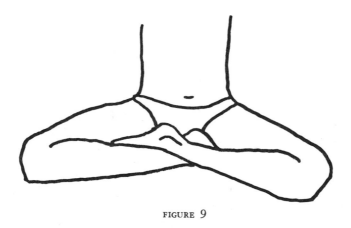

FIGURE 9

(37) Some call this siddhasana; others say it is vajrasana, or muktasana, or guptasana.

Why? Is there a difference of opinion? No, there are good reasons. This asana can serve several purposes, and each name indicates a different emphasis. But we do not want to get lost in details.

*(38) The siddhas say: Just as among the yamas the most impor-
tant is to do no harm to anyone, and that among the niyamas
moderation, so is siddhasana the chief of all asanas.*

We should not take this as a qualitative characteristic. Rather
one should say: just as nonviolence is the leitmotiv of all other
principles, and moderation the guideline to all other qualities, so
also is siddhasana the foundation of all other requirements for
the inner vision of raja yoga (without making them superfluous,
however).

*(39) Of the 84 asanas one should always practice siddhasana
[above all]. It purifies the 72,000 nadis.*

Nadis are those paths through which the body receives its supply
of prana. We should not think of these as nerve strands, and
whether or not there are 72,000 would be hard to ascertain, nor
is it of any consequence. Only three nadis are important for us:
first, the previously mentioned sushumna path in the center of
the spinal column, and then the two major nadis which run
parallel to the spinal column, ida (left) and pingala (right).
   They begin in the nostril of their respective sides, wind once
around the ajna chakra like thread around a spindle, and end all
the way down where the main channel, the sushumna, also ends,
in the muladhara chakra. Since it is the task of these nadis to
circulate the life stream of prana, they must be kept clean, which
is not a simple matter. Under special circumstances this asana
serves the purpose. But there are other methods which are indicated under other conditions. The second part of this work
utilizes them.

*(40) The yogi who meditates on the atman and eats moderately
achieves the yoga siddhis after he has practiced siddhasana for
12 years.*

Atman meditation is reflection upon our own mysterious self; its the way to self-knowledge. God (Brahman) and atman have from time immemorial been the great Oneness: "I am" is the name of God that Moses heard and which is proclaimed as the first name of God in the Jewish Kabbala. It was the same in ancient Egypt and is still so with the Parsis. "I am Brahma" (*brahmasmi*): this is the meditation even of Hindus who are not yogis. Only the meditator, who can experience it, will understand the atman. The intellectual tackles the problem with logic and philosophical deduction which result only in more complications, but will never lead to a solution. Atman meditation is perfect mysticism. As to the 12 years, this is only applicable to the average aspirant. One of my gurus reached his goal in 23 days, but with 16 hours of daily meditation. Had he meditated only eight hours he would perhaps have needed two years, and with four hours probably no less than ten.

(41) If siddhasana is perfected and the breath is carefully restrained in kevala kumbhaka, what need for all the other asanas?

Again a new term, kumbhaka. This is a simple matter: kumbhaka is the moment between inhalation and exhalation, or vice versa, when the breath is retained for some time.

Anyone can observe the development of prana: after a few deep and fast inhalations and exhalations concentrate on the fingertips. What you feel then is the direct effect of prana.

The varieties of kumbhaka, of which kevala kumbhaka is only one, will be discussed later on.

(42) When siddhasana is accomplished, we can enjoy the ecstasy of the meditative state (unmani avastha), the moon and the three bandhas follow without effort naturally.

This sloka is not for the student but for the teacher. The three bandhas are still unknown, the unmani avastha state is a fond hope, and how the moon can "follow" is still a mystery. Have patience; all shall be explained in due course.

(43) There is no asana like siddhasana, no kumbhaka like kevala, no mudra like khecari, and no laya equals nada [anahat nada].

A sloka that the teacher at this point can only underline, while the student hopefully awaits the day when he can convince himself of its efficacy. Whether or not it is valid we can judge only at the end of this book.

(44) Place the right heel upon the base of the left thigh and the left upon the right thigh. Cross the arms behind the back and grasp the toes, the right ones with the right hand and the left with the left. Press the chin on the breast and look at the tip of your nose. This is called padmasana and cures all diseases.* [See Figure 10.]

First of all, it appears that we have here without a doubt a gymnastic exercise of enormous value, but one that demands a high degree of skill. The rib cage is expanded and the lungs and shoulders strengthened, the spinal column is straightened out, and the abdominal muscles stretched: an exemplary posture from a sheer physical point of view.

To this are added deeper results which are immediately manifest when we meditate in this posture. First of all there is completely new awareness of the body; then the spinal column is

---

*"The secret teaching is that there should be a space of four inches between the chin and the breast." Sri Nivasa Iyangar, *The Hatha Yoga Pradipika of Yoga Swami Svatmarama* (translation with commentary) (Adyar, 1949), p. 22. —Trans.

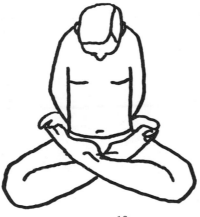

FIGURE 10

reshaped: it becomes straight, whereas usually it is slightly S-shaped; the "kundalini path" is relieved of its curves and thus becomes more readily traversible. But there is also an influence on the chakras, and last but not least, the prana "circuit" is re-channeled. Yet as contradictory as it seems, the value of this asana as a physical exercise is greater than its meditative assets.

Important in this connection is the next asana with the same name, which contains all the benefits that are referred to as secondary in the above asana. The two combined in systematic practice give the results that are desired at this stage of evolution.

(45–47) Place your feet firmly on the opposite thighs and place your hands firmly in the middle, one upon the other [in your lap], fasten your eyes on the tip of the nose and touch the back of the upper teeth with your tongue. Press the chin on the chest and raise the air [apana vayu] slowly up while contracting the anus muscle. This is padmasana that destroys all diseases. [But] this can be achieved by only a few very intelligent persons.

This is the first step to raja yoga. In the previous padmasana we created the essential physical conditions. The spinal column was straightened and the "bow of the nadis" was drawn (as my guru termed it), so that the real yoga could now begin. But even when we have achieved this posture it is like an empty pot, for what is essential here, the prana, will be developed only in the second stage.

This section introduces a part of the anatomy that has not yet been mentioned, as indeed it is not often mentioned: the sphincter muscle of the anus. We should also know that in addition to the prana circuit there are four other similar currents that course through our body, one of which, called apana, flows through the "lower regions," just as prana flows through the respiratory system. We can influence the prana through the process of breathing and the apana through the above-mentioned movement of the sphincter muscle. What for? Again we must look back. It was stated that prana should enter the hairline channel of sushumna; but prana cannot move any lower than the diaphragm, while apana finds its upper boundary below the diaphragm.

If we can "tie" these two streams together, one continuous flow reaches from the nostrils to the end of the spinal cord, thus constituting a single unit able to fulfill its task.

Here the condition has been created that will be utilized practically in the next step.

(48) Having assumed the padmasana posture, with the hands one upon the other, and the chin firmly pressed upon the chest, meditate on Brahma, frequently contracting the anus muscle to raise apana. Similarly, by contracting the throat, force prana down. Thus with the aid of kundalini [which is aroused by this process] we achieve highest knowledge.

*(49) When the yogi remains in padmasana and thus retains the
breath drawn in through the nadi gates [nostrils] he reaches
liberation. There is no doubt about it.*

If everything has been understood thus far, one has an inkling
of what is at stake. Only one point is not quite as clear as it may
sound: that the yogi reaches liberation. Liberation from what?
What is this liberation like?

He is liberated who sees this world for what it really is, a
figment of our own imagination. The nonliberated believed that
he is a part of this tangible world; he has to submit to the
demands of circumstance, and his fortune or misfortune is apparently tied to this tangible world. His desires are for possession
of things or people. He lives only by the consciousness of what
his senses convey to him. And beyond the world of senses there
exists for him only the darkness of dubious fantasies. An uncer-
tain faith in a higher power is about the extent of his other-
worldliness, and more often than not even this is nothing but a
primitive fear of punishment that he expects from someplace
where his earthbound understanding cannot reach. His obedi-
ence to divine laws is based on weakness, not on the recognition
that he himself is a part of that law, a part of the eternal light—
and darkness. These "two souls, alas! in his own breast" chafe
under the material illusion of the cosmos: the insensitive matter
as master of which he entered the world and whose slave he
soon became. He stumbles over the least little stone, curses the
stone, and with his curse strikes only his own weakness. His
condition is hopeless servitude. He who searches for the source
of his sorrow elsewhere, who tries to demolish the stumbling
block without realizing his own unmindfulness, is always a slave.

The liberated one knows and sees all problems within himself.
It is not that he has persuaded himself of this by philosophical

logic. No, he experiences in meditation the forces and the content of his own personality and can objectively oppose them to sense impressions. Once he realizes his true position he is as free from sense impressions as the adult is free from attachment to the toys of his childhood. He views those oh-so-vital things of this world as the grandfather sees the dolls of his grandchildren: not senseless by any means, but not worthy of being idolized at the cost of inner power. To be sure, he cannot persuade the "unfree" child of the "objective uselessness" of the doll with wise words, but under his guidance the child can grow to maturity so that one day she will realize by herself the worthlessness of the doll. Here, similarly, it is useless to try to persuade the average human being of the objective uselessness of his toys as long as he is not ready for it. "Do not show men the real value of their world, but teach them to fathom it for themselves." This is perhaps the aptest tenet in all yoga.

(50) Place your ankles in the region of the sex organs [between anus and scrotum]: the right ankle to the right and the left to the left side.

This means kneel with knees slightly apart, feet crossed. (Compare Fig. 2.)

(51) Place the palms upon the knees with fingers spread out and eyes upon the tip of the nose [and breathe] with open mouth and concentrated mind.

(52) This is simhasana, held in great esteem by the highest yogis. This asana facilitates the three bandhas.

If the student does not know something about the bandhas this asana has little meaning. Bandha comes from "to bind." That there is something to bind we have seen, namely prana (the upper circuit) and apana (the lower circuit).

If we try this asana we realize that the chest expands when we inhale and the abdomen recedes. This is the first step to the bandhas.

(53–55) Place the ankles under the buttocks, right below right, left below left. Then wind your hands around the thighs. This is bhadrasana and cures all diseases. The siddhas and yogis call it gorakshasana. The yogi should practice this until he feels no more pain or tiredness. [See Figure 11.]

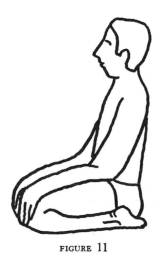

FIGURE 11

Nothing much is gained for raja yoga through this asana. It does control unwanted desires.

(56) Then he should cleanse the nadis by practicing pranayama, as well as mudras and kumbhakas of various kinds.

These will be learned at the next level.

CHAPTER 4

THE WAY OF LIFE OF A YOGI

A FEW useful hints before we attempt the higher goals of the second part. They may not be as dramatic as the slowly clarifying background of asanas, but they are important enough to cause tremendous difficulties if they are ignored.

(57a) Then follows the concentration on the inner sound [nada].

This sloka belongs to the highest form of raja yoga (to be discussed in Part Four), and is rather premature here; it may be an interpolation by an impatient student of Swatmarama.

(57b) The brahmacharin who, observing moderate diet, renouncing the fruits of his actions, practices [hatha] yoga will become a siddha in the span of one year.

A brahmacharin is a yogi who observes complete celibacy. Here the question of celibacy becomes acute. How compulsory is it for a yogi? At this point I cannot give a decisive answer but should say that most of the yoga masters I have known were happy householders, while I have met brahmacharins, on the other hand, who did not distinguish themselves by higher knowledge. It is not as important to withhold potency as it is to know how to manage it and, above all, how to transform it into spiritual potency. Celibacy without transformation of the preserved potencies only forces them to find their own outlet, mostly where it is least desired, at the weakest point of the whole organism.

"Yoga," says my guru, "is economy of forces, not repression of nature." This statement may seem very comforting to some students, but "economy" needs closer definition, for the yogi's "economy" seems like heavy sacrifice to most. Economy of forces means to be in tune with natural harmony. And this is exclusively the measured rhythm of nature. Stimulation does not originate from the outside, artificially, but from inner sources, the essential wellsprings which are within us. It is therefore not a question of overpowering the body or (most curious of all endeavors) of shutting out all the stimuli of the outer world, but a question of illuminating our own consciousness. After that the body obeys automatically. Celibacy of the mind has to precede celibacy of the body. An evil thought is worse than a bad deed.

The "deed in thought" is often underestimated. One imagines control of action is the chief accomplishment, and forgets that frequently lack of opportunity or fear of external laws are the motivations which make us so virtuous. Sigmund Freud has perhaps painted too dark a picture, but we can hardly deny his principle, especially when at a later stage of meditation we are faced with our fearful animalistic self.

Another interesting problem arises from the phrase, "renouncing the fruits of his actions." This is pure karma yoga.

A deed is of value only when it is done for its own sake. This is a platitude which has the remarkable distinction of containing one of the deepest wisdoms of the world. The reason for this and its practical value can easily be explained psychologically but the advantages that result from it internally lie beyond the most fertile imagination. It is easily tested: Anyone who succeeds in doing a really "good deed" without the slightest selfish motive—one of the most difficult tasks a man can accomplish—will reap the joy of its sublime fruit. Everything that we mortals do has a motive, for we are "creatures of reason," and reason always demands the motive (which according to ancient wisdom we are not supposed to have). The psychological explanation for this cannot be discussed here; but whether or not we adopt the path of yoga, we should occasionally analyze one of our "good deeds" to see how much selfishness or self-satisfaction it actually contains. The fruit of every good deed is a certain satisfaction which directly or indirectly results from this deed. And it is this satisfaction that the yogi renounces. He does not create anything in his mind that could be satisfied in this way.

The careful observer will note that the spiritual background of the abstinence of the brahmacharin and the renunciation of the karma yogi have the same source, and that the same psychological disciplines are demanded. There is no doubt that he who can fulfill these conditions can "become a siddha in the span of one year."

Something more has to be said about the "moderate diet":

(58) Moderate diet means pleasant, sweet food, leaving free one fourth of the stomach. The act of eating is dedicated to Siva.

The classical commentary says: "He [the yogi] should fill two parts of his stomach with food, and the third part with water, leaving the fourth free for air to aid the digestive process." In short, moderation.

(59–61) The following are considered as not being salutary: sour, pungent, and hot food; mustard, alcohol, fish, meat, curds, buttermilk,* chick peas, fruit of the jujub, linseed cakes, asafetida, and

---

*This does not refer to the commercially cultured milk we call "buttermilk." —Trans.

garlic. It is also advisable to avoid: reheated food, an excess of salt or acid, foods that are hard to digest or are woody. Gorakṣa teaches that in the beginning the yogi should avoid bad company, proximity to fire, sexual relations, long trips, cold baths in the early morning, fasting, and heavy physical work.

These strict disciplines are imposed on the student, but do not necessarily apply to the master.

"Proximity to fire": the temperature of a yogi changes considerably during specific practices, especially in the meditative state. The term "burning asceticism" (tapas) has its origin here, and is not, as it may seem, sheer rhetoric. If the yogi in training submits to exterior temperature changes through proximity to fire or by a cold bath after the warmth of his couch, he damages through these unnatural changes the "fire of life" (pitta). The temperature of the atmosphere depends on atmospheric pressure, which influences the whole human organism and regulates the pitta. Artificial temperature changes do not agree with the yogi while he is in an altered state. Even the simplest practice of meditation becomes senseless if the yogi is freezing. This is one of the reasons why the coverings of a kundalini yogi consist always of silk or wool, never of cotton [or manmade fibers —Trans.].

(62) The following items can be used without hesitation: wheat products [bread, etc.] rice, milk, fats, rock candy, honey, dried ginger, cucumbers, vegetables, and fresh water.

(63) The yogi should eat nourishing, sweet foods mixed with milk. They should benefit the senses and stimulate the functions.

(64) Anyone who actively practices yoga, be he young, old, or even very old, sickly or weak, can become a siddha.

(65) Anyone who practices can acquire siddhis, but not he who is lazy. Yoga siddhis are not obtained by merely reading textbooks.

(66) Nor are they reached by wearing yoga garments or by conversation about yoga, but only through tireless practice. This is the secret of success. There is no doubt about it.

(67) The various asanas, kumbhakas, and mudras of hatha yoga should be practiced as long as raja yoga has not been attained.

And when will that have been attained? When human existence no longer holds any problems.

PART TWO

THE RIVER OF LIFE

CHAPTER 5

THE PURIFICATION OF THE NADIS

AFTER the broad outline of the evolution of the whole organism through asanas given in Part One, we come to the vata element in all its aspects. Only he can grasp the deepest sense of pranayama who is open-minded enough to view each concept in three dimensions: gross (physical), subtle (mental), and abstract (spiritual); or dynamic, static, and abstract. When he recognizes the interrelation of these aspects, he may come to that cognition which converts the wisdom of yoga into revelation.

(1) When the yogi has perfected his asanas he should practice pranayama according to the instructions of his master. With controlled senses he should nourish himself with moderation.

At a higher level of instruction things begin to change in many ways. The guru is not as lenient as in the beginning. He gives higher initiation and a new mantra (more about this later), speaks less, expects more. Perhaps not yet in achievement, but in terms of understanding. Nor does he like to refer back to the first level of practice. We too will find that recapitulation is seldom needed.

(2) When the breath "wanders" [i.e., is irregular] the mind also is unsteady. But when the breath is calmed, the mind too will be

71

still, and the yogi achieves long life. Therefore, one should learn to control the breath.

Have you ever noticed how the breath becomes irregular on certain occasions? Certainly, if you try to catch a bus you breathe irregularly afterwards and are fully aware of the fact that you are "out of breath." But that is not what I mean.

Take for example two other occasions: in the theater, and at an important interview. How was your breathing in the first instance and how in the second? When was it slower, when faster? When was it regular? And how was it when it was irregular? Thus one could ask a thousand questions on a thousand occasions and receive a thousand different replies—if the interviewed person knew anything about his breath. But he knows nothing about his breath and therefore knows nothing about his mind. This conclusion is incontrovertible.

Certainly we may know this or that about our thoughts—for instance, what we have been thinking of—but do we know why we thought just about this and not about anything else? We know that suddenly another thought arose, but do not know the relationship between the two thoughts. We know that we remember certain things easily and forget others quite readily, but why? It is just the thing behind this "why" that is the most important part of our mind. It is the source of our mental existence.

Still the question of the relationship of mind with breath remains unresolved. Here we could marshal many formulas which have physiological foundations, such as oxygen supply, heart rhythm, blood circulation, blood supply to the brain cells. But all these are not decisive factors. What is decisive is what is only imperfectly understood: the significance of the lifestream or prana as power source of our thought creator, "mind."

All these are ponderous and complicated problems, but let us simply mention them here. Later slokas will lead us closer to a solution, at least as close as it is necessary for a yogi at the second stage of training. So let us advance cautiously on this shaky ground.

(3) Man lives only as long as he has breath in his body. If he lacks breath [prana] he dies. Therefore we should practice prana-yama.

We know, of course, that breath is life; we even know the chemical process that proves it. But how is it that we cannot keep a dying man alive by attaching him to an oxygen tank? So it is not just oxygen that matters. Is the decisive element the life-stream, prana?

(4) When the nadis are impure, breath cannot penetrate into the sushumna. Then the yogi achieves nothing, nor can he reach the state of deep concentration [unmani avastha].

We know that 72,000 nadis in our body are the conveyors of the life current, and that we live our everyday lives by this current. The higher life of a yogi is achieved by creating an additional supply of current to send through the otherwise weakly supplied main channel (sushumna). This causes heightened activities in the chakras and brain centers, resulting in the yogi's higher state of consciousness. It is well known that a rusty conductor uses more power than a clean one. Similarly, if the nadis are impure, pranayama is a waste of energy.

(5) Only when all the nadis which are still impure are purified can the yogi practice pranayama successfully.

(6) Therefore one should practice pranayama with the mind in sattvic condition until the sushumna is free from impurities.

73

There are two methods of purification of the nadis. Here we describe the psychological method which is far more pleasant than the other, although the second one leads more speedily to the goal.

One should practice "with the mind in a sattvic state." We shall try to understand this without burdening the mind with the intricacies of the guna theory.

Sattva is the positive propensity for purity. Good deeds, kind words, noble thoughts, a pleasing personality, interest in lofty pursuits are the distinguishing marks of sattva. And remember, it is not the activity that is decisive. One single impure thought during pranayama and the current is disturbed; not only the current but the whole being, since a human being becomes a human being only by this electromagnetic current.

We can readily imagine how this can happen: we perceive something; it is carried on the life stream to the brain, as a live reflex. So far we can call it "the pure idea." Once it reaches thinking it is already colored by the personality and has thus become individualized. It is then evaluated; and this again is entirely individual. If in addition it is then stained by an impure mind, our whole personality is contaminated.

These seemingly trivial impurities are still coarse enough to block the psychic pathway of the nadis. This statement would be absurd if the nadis were what they are not, bodily organs. Rather they are magnetic fields, such as are developed by a magnet.

If we now become aware that every breath we take is in a sense pranayama, we can readily realize how frequently we damage our delicate psyche with an impure or bad thought. In the long run we shorten our lives with every negative gesture in deed, word, or thought by overburdening the conductors of the life stream with these impurities.

(7) Assuming the padmasana posture, the yogi shall guide the prana through the left nostril [chandra = moon] *to the ida nadi, and, after having retained the breath as long as possible* [in kumbhaka], *should exhale it through the right nostril* [surya = sun].

(8) Then he should inhale through the right nostril, do kumbhaka according to the rule, and exhale through the left nostril.

(9) Inhalation is [always] *through the same nostril as the previous exhalation. After the breath has been retained to the utmost possible limit* [until perspiration breaks out or the body begins to tremble], *one should exhale slowly—never quickly* [since that reduces the energy of the body].

(10) Take in prana through the ida nadi and exhale it through the pingala. Then take in [new prana] *through pingala and release it through ida, after having held it* [in kumbhaka] *as long as possible. The yogi who has perfected himself in the yamas* [having thus developed the sattvic mind] *will purify his nadis in three months* [of practice].

This is the technique of pranayama. Just as all the multitude of asanas aim at the spinal column, so the essence of prana is centered in kumbhaka, the period when there is no breathing. From this as well as by later indications we can recognize that it is not the breath air that carries the current but that the current is being produced during the breathing process.

Just as the plunging waters in a power plant are only the means of releasing the energy through which the brushes of the stationary turbines are activated, so prana also does not originate in breath but in the "turbins," the chakra wheels with which the nadis have an inductive relationship.

The current necessary to sustain our life is automatically regulated through the varying strength of our inhalation and exhalation. Sighing and yawning are pranayamas in miniature but with different purposes. Our critical medico will patronizingly tell us that yawning and sighing are functions that regulate the oxygen supply in our blood. True. We do not try to belittle this fact. And we know that physiologically the production of electromagnetic current is so minimal as to be barely measurable: a negligible factor, just as one hundred years ago the microscopic secretions of the endocrine glands were considered negligible. But man is more than a chemical laboratory, and we have no right to designate even the slightest manifestations as unimportant until we have proof.

We should, therefore, not be surprised at the yogis' contention that the heart is not the most important organ of man. It is the power centers, though they have not yet been seen by anyone, that are most vital. The heart is a muscle and becomes a regulator of bodily functions only in relation to and in cooperation with other organs, while these invisible centers supervise and guide the organs because they are directly subordinate to the mind.

(11) Four times a day we should practice kumbhaka: early morning, midday, evening, and midnight, until we can do 80 rounds [at a time].

A commentary speaks of three phases: at the beginning the breath should be held for 30 seconds, at the second stage for 60 seconds, and at the third for 90 seconds.

(12) At the first stage perspiration breaks out, at the second stage the body trembles, and at the third stage prana reaches

76

the center of the head by way of sushumna. In this way prana-
yama should be practiced.

This may sound rather violent, but do not forget that the main characteristic of yoga is not violence but perseverance, not compulsion but patience. However, there is a limit beyond which perseverance becomes pigheadedness and patience apathy. The yogi has to recognize and respect these limits. This is one of the most difficult tasks in his whole career. Proof: take one of the more difficult asana and try to hold it longer than your physical forces can naturally allow. The signs of violence and undue constraint, perspiration and trembling, will appear; heavy breathing and tightening of the lips will also testify to a conflict. One fights against one's own self. One part wants to stop; the other to continue. These manifestations are signs of undue force; it is quite different when perseverance and patience are at play without any compulsion. But for this we need a certain noncompulsive way of practice that is the leitmotiv of the whole yoga system. It is difficult to learn from books and only the guru can show us the true path: meditative practice.

The half-trained yogi pays attention primarily to the body when doing the asanas, i.e., to the various positions of the limbs that he wants to place into the prescribed pose. And this is a gross mistake. He should concentrate on the "asana as such," less on its physical manifestation, and far less on the body that moves and gets into postures. The less conscious attention the yogi pays to his body the more perfect will be his asana. If the phrase "asana as such" seems strange to us, this indicates that we have not yet fathomed the deeper essence of asanas, their really great meaning.

In order to show you that asanas are more than consciously created gymnastic exercises, let me describe a mysterious manifestation that is usually witnessed only by the initiated. The process, called kriyavati, manifests in yogis who have awakened kundalini by way of hatha yoga.

The yogi sits in deep meditation. Breath is suspended, the body is cold and stiff. Only the topmost center of his skull is feverishly hot.

Then he starts moving his limbs. An inner mechanism seems to be at work. Slowly, steadily, with unencumbered ease his arms intertwine, the legs go into contortions, the spinal column twists: asanas perfected to the utmost. He includes asanas no textbook has ever described; the guhyasanas, positions that are imparted to the student orally only after certain initiations. They are asanas that can be performed only by the yogi who has learned to govern his body completely with his higher consciousness.

The yogi does not perform these asanas in waking consciousness. "It" performs the asanas in him, while his waking state has yielded completely to a state beyond the borderline of perception.

In this state the yogi is capable of superhuman physical achievements. Thus we find in Tibet the lunggompas, yogis who in a meditative state cover hundreds of miles with great speed. Dizzying precipices and snowstorms cannot hinder their course, much less stop them. Attempts to follow on a galloping horse have always failed. No horse has ever passed this prodigious test.

In this state there is no trembling, no perspiring. This is one of the higher forms of yoga; we are still working on a considerably lower level. The ideal we are now aspiring to lies halfway between our usual awareness of bodily movement and the kriyavati state. The ebbing of physical strength during practice manifests by trembling and perspiration; consciousness remains calm and relaxed. The mind, not burdened with any feeling of compulsion to persist, rests in itself, in the "asana as such." This is the essential difference.

So when here on the first level perspiration breaks out, this is a sign of compulsion only if consciousness occupies itself with this fact. If the mind remains calm, there is no thought of compulsion.

(13) Massage the perspiring body. This imparts lightness and strength to the whole constitution.

(14) At the beginning of practice the yogi should nourish himself with milk and ghee [clarified butter]. When he is advanced such restrictions are no longer needed.

(15) Just as lions, elephants, and tigers are tamed [little by little, with patience and energy], so the prana should be kept under control. Otherwise it can kill the practicer.

(16) By the practice of pranayama we deliver ourselves from all diseases. By faulty practice the yogi invites all kinds of ailments.

(17) Then breath takes a wrong course and practice results in coughs, asthma, headaches, eye and ear pain, as well as other sicknesses.

The classical example of wrong practice is told of Ramakrishna, the famous nineteenth-century saint. In his youth his practice invariably ended in a blackout. Later bloodshot eyes and bleeding of the gums developed, and the end result of this faulty practice was cancer of the throat, of which he died. His saintliness was not the result of this type of practice; but self-destructive extremism is an indication of the kind of ruthlessness man is capable of.

(18) Slowly one should inhale and exhale, and proceed gradu ally also with kumbhaka. Thus one will attain the siddhis.

(19) When the nadis are purified, certain signs quite naturally manifest: the body becomes light and bright.

(20) As soon as the nadis are purified the yogi is able to retain the breath longer, the gastric fire is activated, nada [the inner sound] becomes audible and he enjoys perfect health.

Perfect health alone is reason enough to concern ourselves with nadi purification. About the gastric fire and the nada sound we will learn more later. But it is the art of retention of breath that is so essential in the development of pranayama.

How is it that the power to hold the breath for a considerable length of time should depend on the purity of the nadis rather than on the capacity of the lungs?

Breath gets short when the air held in the lungs has lost its prana. If the nadis are impure (as is common), then the flow of prana is impeded and is soon unable to reload the breath. The breath becomes stale like a carbonated drink when it has lost its fizz. If the nadi path is pure, however, the prana flow can keep breath "alive" for a longer time.

A yogi who can subsist on one breath for days—as has been demonstrated—causes the river of prana to circulate in the body and does not allow the prana to escape. He absorbs oxygen through his pores.

Now let us look at the technique of nadi purification.

(21) He who is of weak constitution and phlegmatic, subject to kapha disorders, should first practice shatkarma. Those not suf fering [constitutionally] from the [main] disorders due to vata, pitta, and kapha do not need it.

The nadis of all students, even the healthiest, need purifying. The man of perfect health, the sportsman, the master of asanas whose physical training is nearer perfection than his mental-spiritual achievement can reach nadi perfection by cultivating the mental-spiritual aspect. For the one who first must think of physical-organic purification because he senses problems and shortcomings, shatkarma (the "sixfold activity") is indicated.

(22) Shatkarma is dhauti, vasti, neti, trataka, nauli, and kapalabhati.

(23) These six practices, which cleanse the body, should be carefully kept secret because they induce numerous wonderful results and are therefore held in high esteem with the great yogis.

Why this secretiveness? What are these "wonderful results"?

Imagine a man who uses a low-tension electrical gadget, which is attached by a transformer to high-power current. The current he uses is barely noticeable with the fingertips. With the transformer removed he receives an electric shock.

Exactly so is it here. The unclean nadis act as a transformer to the life stream so that nothing untoward can happen. When the nadis are clean the effectiveness of prana is many times increased, and this can become dangerous.

(24–25) Take a strip of clean cloth, four fingers broad and 15 spans long and slowly swallow it as instructed by the guru. Then pull it back out. This is dhauti and is effective against asthma, illness of the pancreas, leprosy, and other diseases due to kapha.

(26–28) Sit in a tub of water so as to be submerged up to the navel, in crouching position, heels pressed against the buttocks.

Introduce a thin bamboo pipe into the anus, contract the anus muscle [to draw in the water] and move the water around inside. This is vasti and cures troubles of the spleen, edema, and other ailments that are due to an oversupply of vata, pitta, and kapha. This vasti, when properly practiced, refines the circulation of the body fluids, the function of the senses and the heart. It makes the body bright and increases the gastric fire. All constitutional defects are [thus] removed.

So much ado about a simple enema! If this simple remedy is a golden treasure in the West, how much greater must its value be in the tropics. It is a common procedure. Gandhi always practiced it.

All this of course without pranayama. When that is added the whole picture changes and greatest caution is indicated.

(29–30) Pull a thread, 12 inches in length, through one of the nostrils and let its end emerge through the mouth. This is neti. It cleanses the skull and makes the eyes sharp. It also removes illnesses that are above the shoulders.

It certainly is not an agreeable feeling to push a wet cord through the nostrils and let it come out in the back of the throat, picking it up with two fingers and pulling it back and forth through the nostril. But actually it is much more disagreeable to watch the procedure than it is to do it. The yogi himself gets used to it, and is happily free from colds and sinus trouble.

(31–32) Gaze without blinking [with concentrated mind] on a small object, until tears come into your eyes. This is called trataka by the gurus. Trataka cures all diseases of the eyes and removes tiredness. Therefore it should be carefully kept secret, like a treasure box.

Here one senses an ulterior motive. The practice must be kept secret, just because it trains the eyes? This can hardly be the real reason. There actually is a much more plausible reason to observe secrecy.

Hypnosis, self-hypnosis, visions, trance states, ecstasies, hallucinations—these are things that have always seemed very attractive. Everyone would like to experience something like that without endangering himself. And this practice leads exactly in that direction. One could call it false meditation. From the point of view of yoga, all phenomena related to hypnosis are completely useless if not downright dangerous. The premature experimenter invariably draws the wrong conclusions from his experiences. The real meditative states are cognitive, clear consciousness. There are no surprise manifestations. This practice (tratakam) is salutary if done with proper care. It is poison if forced too fast.

(33-34) With head bent forward slowly rotate the innards [intestines and stomach], like a whirlpool in a river, toward the right and toward the left. This the siddhas call nauli. This, the most important of all hatha yoga practices, removes sluggishness of the gastric fire, stimulates digestion, and leaves a very agreeable feeling. It removes all diseases.

This practice belongs not only to shatkarma but also to regular hatha yoga, although it cannot be called an asana since asana means "position, seat," a motionless posture, while nauli is a movement of the abdominal muscles. In shatkarma it is rather a subsidiary, as it trains the muscles for dhauti and basti. This practice—which is to be recommended to the obese—begins with deep exhalation. At the same time, lean forward with hands pressed on the thighs and draw in the abdomen while raising the shoulders; then try to tighten the drawn-in abdominal muscles. Once this is accomplished the circular motion is no problem, since the muscles stand out separately on the withdrawn abdomen, as thick as a child's arm.

(35) Inhale and exhale like the bellows of a blacksmith. This is kapalabhati and removes all ailments due to kapha.

(36) One frees oneself from obesity and phlegm by these six practices, and is successful if one adds pranayama after them.

Yet it is more advisable to follow the mental method of nadi purification, because progress and purification then go hand in hand. Besides:

(37) Some teachers say that all impurities can be removed through pranayama alone, with nothing else.

And those teachers who say it must know what they are talking about. Shatkarma is a gross physical method, while pranayama purification, completely founded on the sattvic mind, represents an all-encompassing purification. Shatkarma is the purification of the lower stages of hatha yoga, while pranayama belongs to the higher form of yoga, raja yoga.

The following practice does not belong to shatkarma. True, it has the characteristics of shatkarma, but something else is involved.

(38) Closing the sphincter muscle at the anus, draw up apana toward the throat and regurgitate what is in the stomach. In this way the nadi chakras are brought under control. This is gajakarani.

If we remember the counter current to prana, apana in the abdomen, we know that this current cannot move beyond the diaphragm. It is impossible to bring it to the throat. But one can—and should, in this case—cause the apana current to press against the udana current, the current of digestion in the upper part of the abdomen. This is what causes regurgitation.

As previously mentioned we are not really dealing with a purification process here, since dhauti has already done its work. Rather, we stimulate the nervous system directly by the effort of regurgitation.

But just as today's yogis do not advocate this type of practice so we too will leave it alone, as this sutra clearly seems to be a much later interpolation.

After these more or less agreeable purification practices we return to pranayama.

(39) Brahma and the other gods who devoted themselves to the practice of pranayama delivered themselves [by it] from fear of death. This is why we [too] should practice it.

(40) When the breath is controlled, the mind firm and unshakable, the eyes fastened between the eyebrows; why then should we fear death?

Even a man who—like the yogi—has to fear no punishment at the last judgment approaches his last moments with at least some apprehension, for the process of dying is beyond our sphere of control. Here, for better or worse, we are delivered over to the play of natural forces, and this is for man the most terrifying experience: to be a helpless victim.

For the master of pranayama, things are different. He controls the powers that represent life. He dies consciously. In life as in death he adapts himself with deep insight to the natural processes of which he is always aware. It is not only the life stream of prana upon which preservation and end depend, for if

85

such were the case the yogi would be immortal. Rather, he recognizes the rhythm to which he, like all other living things, is subject, and it is his task to gain the highest possible harmony with this rhythm. Once he has accomplished this and his cycle of existence is completed, he will not try to influence the law of his sunset. This death for him is only the evening which is followed by a new and purer morning, a new cycle. It is said to be one of the characteristics of the gods that they have no fear of death to which they are subject like all living things, because they consciously enter the eternally new cycle of life and consciously pass through the transitory, purifying state of death. Again and again Vishnu passes through existence: as animal, man, hero, lover, dwarf, or giant. He is born, accomplishes his divine work, dies, and is reborn. His consciousness is the all-preserving Unconscious.

To render this Unconscious conscious is the goal of the yoga master, for this is the only way to become equal to the gods. So let us too pay attention to the physical and spiritual purity of the nadis, whether or not we are yogis. Let us inhale the life stream without weighing it down with impure thoughts. Let us also live more consciously, with our inner vision concentrated on that which elevates us above all other creatures: our spirit. Then every breath is pranayama which makes us more divine.

(41) As soon as the nadis have been purified through systematic pranayama, breath easily finds its way to the sushumna entrance.

(42) When breath flows through the sushumna, mind becomes steady. This steadiness of the mind is called unmani avastha.

(43) To attain this the sage practices a variety of kumbhakas whereby he acquires siddhis.

CHAPTER 6

KUMBHAKA

WHEN we now speak of the various forms of kumbhaka you should not try to understand it all at once in the first few sentences. Everything that follows is so important that some details have to be made clear first. So do not let your thoughts race away; whatever is not explained now will be discussed later on.

(44) There are eight kumbhakas: suryabhedana, ujjayi, sitkari, sitali, bhastrika, bhramari, murccha and plavini.

(45) At the end of inhalation [puraka] one should do jalandhara bandha; and at the end of kumbhaka and the beginning of exhalation [recaka] uddiyana bandha should be done.

How does this work out in practice? The yogi sits cross-legged on the floor, hands on knees, and inhales deeply. Then he holds his breath, with chin pressed against the chest, abdomen withdrawn. This is jalandhara-bandha.

As soon as his breath is short he raises the head and exhales as deeply as possible. When he has reached the limit he again holds his breath, straightens up the body and draws in the abdomen, whereby a pressure is created on the stomach area, which is increased when he again presses the chin against the chest.

The first part of the practice (inhalation and jalandhara

bandha) concerns the upper half of the spinal column, the "moon"; the second part (exhalation and uddiyana bandha) involves the "sun" in the center of the body (solar plexus). But something else is added, as the next sutra tells us:

(46) When at the same time the throat is contracted and mula-bandha practiced [i.e., the sphincter of the anus is contracted], breath flows through the sushumna, driven by [the pressure exerted by] the navel region [at the time of exhalation].

Anyone who tries this practice and thinks he has succeeded in guiding the breath through the sushumna had better remember the purity of the nadis; with the second attempt, he should become aware how tense he is during this practice. The purpose of the asanas as taught in Part One is to train the body so that no unnecessary exertion will deplete the extra prana supply that has been acquired. It is not sufficient to install the wiring and have proper outlets; it is also necessary to have current in proper voltage and amperes. Otherwise the result is either no light at all or a short circuit. We must be especially careful to avoid the latter; for human "fuses" cannot be replaced.

(47) By contracting the anus [to force apana] upward and forcing prana down from the throat, the yogi becomes a youth of 16 years and is forever free from old age.

Or, stating it more modestly: he who succeeds in uniting the two main currents in the body will thereby eliminate the causes of premature old age. The most significant of these causes is the lack of utilization of the body's natural regenerative powers. Here, two limited main currents are combined that complement each other; together they accomplish what they cannot do singly. Prana and apana are "knotted" in the navel area (nabhi granthi), creating an aggregate that gives youthful strength to the aging yogi. This is the first step in raja yoga.

Once again, the main part of pranayama is kumbhaka, and this can be performed in various ways.

(48) Sitting down comfortably in a good asana, the yogi should inhale through the right nostril.

*(49) [Then] he should do kumbhaka until he feels that the whole body from head to toes is suffused by prana; then he should slowly exhale through the left nostril.**

(50) This suryabheda kumbhaka should be practiced again and again for it cleanses the brain [forebrain and sinuses], *destroys intestinal worms and all the diseases that arise from an over- abundance of vata* [wind].

This is the first and the most commonly practiced of the eight varieties of kumbhaka. We should also note that before we begin this practice we exhale deeply.

(51–52) With closed mouth inhale deeply until the breath fills all the space between the throat and the heart (i.e., to the tips of the lungs). This creates a noise. Do kumbhaka and exhale through the left nostril. This removes phlegm in the throat and enhances the digestive power of the body. This is ujjayi and can be practiced walking or sitting. It keeps diseases away from the individual organs and the nadis, especially diseases that are due to kapha.

*"This is to be done alternately with both nostrils, drawing in through the one and expelling through the other." Pancham Sinh, *Hatha Yoga Pradipika* (translation with commentary) (Allahabad, 1915), p. 21

The noise mentioned is a special characteristic of this kumbhaka. It occurs in a perfectly natural way. We know that with straight body we should exhale deeply before each kumbhaka. During the short pause made after exhalation, when the abdominal wall is drawn inward, the glottis invariably closes. Inhalation through both nostrils simultaneously will cause the glottis to open abruptly; thus ensues the noise.

This kumbhaka seems to deal with the body onesidedly, for while we inhale through both nostrils at the same time, we exhale through the left only. This, of course, makes no difference to the lungs, but all the more to the nadis, and here the heart is especially involved. And that the heart is heavily influenced we can ascertain after the first round. Ujjayi kumbhaka should be practiced only by those whose heart is completely sound; otherwise it can lead to complications.

What is the special benefit of this kumbhaka, apart from its therapeutic influence on kapha? The heart rhythm does not function by itself. It is the pacemaker of all other bodily functions. In yoga it is sometimes necessary to change certain rhythms, and this is one of a number of methods. The organic rhythm is much too important a function to be subjected to willful experiments. The guru knows its meaning and purpose.

(53–55) With tongue protruding a little between the lips, draw in the breath through the mouth with a hissing sound [after kumbhaka]: *exhale through the nose. This is sitkari. By repeating this, the yogi becomes beautiful as a god. All women admire him; he is in control of his actions and feels no hunger, thirst, or fatigue. He gains physical strength and becomes master of yoga, free from all dangers.*

Obviously an enticing practice, and not even a dangerous one if one does not overdo it, as is so often the case with enticements.

We should, however, not be disappointed if we do not activate a love charm, but simply fan the pitta (the "fire of life") to heightened activity. We have already seen what benefits this brings in its wake, and here we should not expect anything further.

(56–57) With tongue protruding still further, inhale. Then follows kumbhaka and exhalation through the nose. This kumbhaka, called sitali, removes illnesses of the spleen, fever, gall bladder trouble, hunger, thirst, and the effects of poison, as for example snake bites.

Here again the therapeutic purpose concerns pitta, but the practice has also another purpose. He who succeeds in inhaling and exhaling deeply with protruding tongue without having his stomach turn will feel that the breath follows an unusual path, for it gets into the stomach. And what happens there?

We remember that the countercurrent to prana is apana in the abdomen. The alert reader will long have wondered: If we must do so much breathing to acquire the extra prana how do we get the corresponding quantity of apana for the abdomen? For what accumulated there has long been washed out by vasti. Sitali is the practice that corrects this deficiency.

(58-60) Place the feet on the [opposite] *thighs. This is padmasana and removes all diseases. Having assumed this posture, exhale with closed mouth until a pressure is felt on the heart, the throat and the head. Then one draws in the breath with a hissing sound until it touches the heart. During all this time head and body are kept straight.*

(61–62) Again inhale and exhale as indicated, again and again, as a blacksmith works his bellows. In this way the prana is kept

in constant circulation in the body. When tired exhale through the right nostril. This is bhastrika kumbhaka.

There are two variations of the same pranayama, one slow, the other fast. It becomes most effective when both kinds are combined in one sitting. With too intensive practice, colored flames dance before the eyes and a blackout is imminent.

In this practice of pranayama the body becomes saturated with prana—in fact, it becomes so "overloaded" that even the inexperienced student can feel the prana. After about five rounds of the "bellows," hold the breath. What then becomes palpable in the fingertips is prana. After a little practice, this current on one's skin can even be felt by another person.

(63–64) When the breath flows through the body, close the nose with thumb, ringfinger [and little finger —Trans.]. Having then performed kumbhaka according to the rule, exhale through the left nostril. This removes illnesses caused by an overabundance of pitta, kapha, and vata, and stimulates the gastric fire of the body.

Through this bhastrika kumbhaka alone it is not possible for the breath to penetrate the whole body. However, when we combine the protruding-tongue practice described above with the "bellows"—in the sequence mentioned—then this actually does happen. And with this another important step has been taken in the direction of the sleeping kundalini serpent.

(65) Thus kundalini rises quickly, the nadis are purified, it is pleasant, and of all kumbhakas the most beneficial. In this manner phlegm at the mouth of the sushumna is removed.

The procedure is as follows: In sitali kumbhaka the body is filled with apana. In bhastrika kumbhaka the necessary amount of prana is created, and then for the first time, the two currents are brought to face each other. Through jalandhara bandha, uddiyana bandha, and mula bandha, these two currents are knotted together (nabhi granthi) and now raja yoga can begin.

(66) Bhastrika kumbhaka should be practiced especially, for it forces the breath to pierce the three knots that are in the sushumna.

Although the "three knots" (Brahma granthi, Vishnu granthi, and Rudra granthi) are extremely significant, we shall give here only a short theoretical survey.

The three stations of human evolution ("focusing, unfolding, and change" [Rousselle], or the "via purgativa, via illuminativa, via unitiva" of the Christian mystic) are directly dependent on the three knots, which in the process of higher evolution have to be pierced. Each breakthrough is accompanied by a catharsis, which here, in kundalini yoga, also manifests on a physical level. [See Part One, Slokas 27-28 —Trans.]

We have now learned the essentials. The propitious exterior conditions have been established, the necessary asanas carefully practiced; and through proper pranayama the channels of prana, the nadis, have been purified. This is the first step to raja yoga. Then we began the "production" of prana:

1. By alternate inhalation and exhalation, left and right (surya bheda kumbhaka), prana was created.
2. Then the muscles of the throat and the anus sphincter were trained (bandhas).
3. The heart was then prepared for the heavy work ahead (ujjayi kumbhaka).
4. The volume of the lungs was increased (sitkari kumbhaka).
5. We learned the art of guiding the breath into the abdominal cavity (sitali kumbhaka).

6. There then followed the first serious attempt to test what had been learned (bhastrika kumbhaka).

At this point we have accomplished a great deal, but we are still far from the goal. Once the yogi has experienced what he has learned on this level of training, his real work can begin. To become a master in pranayama is simply a question of perseverance, patience and endless effort.

A few special pranayamas follow which should not be confused with the others.

(67) Inhale rapidly, producing the sound of a male bee. Then exhale with the sound of a female bee. This is followed by kumbhaka. The great yogis, by constantly practicing this, experience indescribable happiness in their hearts. This is bhramari.

A strange kumbhaka for which there are many reasons, the most profound of which we will learn in Part Four. Whether or not we imitate a bee successfully is of minor importance. Essential is the humming sound which should be accompanied by concentrated inward vision. If the nadis are pure and there is no muscle tension, the humming inhalation brings with it the sense that one is absorbing something tangible (something that expresses itself in the sound) and thereby dissolving it. Kumbhaka then follows, accompanied by an extraordinary, suspended, potentially filled silence. Now exhalation follows—the longest process timewise—and here the humming becomes an experience. The vibrating sound seems to become a rushing noise that fills the whole atmosphere. A whole world seems to emerge, fashioned completely from vibrations. It becomes stronger and stronger until one is tempted to open the eyes, as one cannot imagine that this roaring sound exists only in one's own body. If one remains steady and does not yield to this desire to open the eyes, then that feeling of happiness occurs, a feeling as though one had just witnessed an extraordinary natural phenomenon whereby one was allowed a glimpse into the divine workshop. One is convinced that with these vibrations one could tumble down whole buildings, that one could change the very structure of objects, as though . . . but now the breath is ended and it again becomes as strangely still as before. But this is not the calm of great expectations; it is the calm after the battle, still echoing with threats. When now the humming inhalation follows, a whole world seems to crumble. Everything one has built up disintegrates in a short, rough, seemingly cruel and hideous process.

Thus the pendulum swings from breath to breath, from creation to dissolution and from there back to creation again. Whether all this can happen without the influence of the guru is hard to say. My guru practiced along with me at first and then gradually dropped back without my noticing it.

In principle we have here the essence of a whole yoga system. He who has grasped the deeper sense of this kumbhaka and its related phenomena has saved himself years of study. One thing, of course, must be understood: he has knowledge, but he is not yet a master.

(68) At the end of inhalation do jalandhara bandha and then slowly exhale. This is murccha kumbhaka. It causes a kind of stupor of the mind and is very agreeable.

This kumbhaka too has its peculiarities, which even the text itself recognizes.

We recall the jalandhara bandha (Part Two, 45), which—please note this—comes usually at the end of exhalation. Here it is reversed, and we recognize the many-sided character of this kind of practice. Here the purpose differs widely from our

95

previous method, for now we have to learn to execute a practice while the observing mind disappears. That is, we are to study (in relative safety) the moment of consciously induced unconsciousness.

The strange trance state (to be discussed later) is, of course, not an unconscious state in the ordinary sense; rather it is extremely heightened consciousness, concentrated on a single point in which all else disappears. In other words, it is an unconscious state, generally speaking, but it is more precisely a heightened consciousness. Now the yogi must learn to recognize the image of the transitory stage, of the razor's edge between the superconscious and the unconscious. If he makes the slightest mistake later and falls from the superconscious into the unconscious state of a faint it can mean death or insanity. Here he is learning to anaesthetize discursive thinking without becoming unconscious; he has also not yet awakened the powerful force of kundalini.

(69) Having filled the lungs completely with air, the yogi floats upon the water like a lotus leaf. This is plavini kumbhaka.

Nothing else is mentioned. Nothing about health or long life, only a rather extravagant-sounding promise. For we all know, regardless of how deeply we inhale, we will hardly float along like a lotus leaf, no more easily, in any case, than we are used to in swimming.

Since this kumbhaka, though useful, is not in any way decisive, we shall only comment briefly: his body having been emptied completely through the much-debated process of shatkarma, the yogi fills all the cavities with air: lungs, stomach, intestines. Thus the "floating like a lotus leaf" becomes more plausible.

So much for the eight varieties of pranayama. A few general remarks will close this subject.

(70) There are three kinds of pranayamas: Recaka pranayama (exhalation), puraka pranayama (inhalation) and kumbhaka pranayama (retention). Kumbhaka is also of two kinds: sahita and kevala.

The types of prana are summarized:

1. Prana that results from kumbhaka after exhalation.
2. Prana that originates from kumbhaka after inhalation.
3. Prana that is developed
   a. through holding the breath at any time and any place, without force or exertion (sahita)
   b. by holding the breath when the blood is overoxygenized (kevala).

(71) As long as one has not yet [fully] mastered kevala kumbhaka, which means holding the breath without inhalation or exhalation, one should practice sahita.

(72–73) When kevala kumbhaka without inhalation and exhalation has been mastered, there is nothing in the [inner] world that is unattainable for the yogi. Through this kumbhaka he can restrain the breath as long as he likes.

(74–75) Thus he [gradually] attains the stage of raja yoga. Through this kumbhaka, kundalini is aroused and then the sushumna is free from all obstacles; but without hatha yoga there can be no raja yoga, and vice versa. Both should be practiced until raja yoga is perfected.

(76) At the end of kumbhaka he should withdraw his mind from all objects. By doing this regularly he reaches raja yoga.

(77) *The signs of perfection in hatha yoga are: a lithe body, harmonious speech, perception of the inner sound (nada), clear eyes, health, controlled seminal flow, increased gastric fire, and purity of the nadis.*

And thus equipped the yogi can confidently embark upon the third stage of his training, where new, greater and more decisive things are awaiting him.

PART THREE

ACTIVE YOGA

CHAPTER 7

THE MUDRAS

(1) Just as Ananta the lord of the serpents [the "infinite one" with seven heads] supports the whole universe with its mountains and woods, even so is kundalini the mainstay of all yoga practices.

The leitmotiv is majestically clear here. We are entering into the inner sanctum of the secret temple. Now the preparatory work is completed; things are called by their real names, and yet—: this "master," who now sees with open eyes what is at stake, suddenly becomes aware that he is still only a student. The master of pranayama is a lesser master, for he still has to prove himself. He does not even suspect yet that some day he will have to forget all that he has learned in the course of many years; he does not suspect that all these wonderful experiences are dangerous reefs that imperil his way to the highest abstract knowledge. If he knew all this now he would be troubled by doubts or would try to reach what he is not yet capable of finding. Nature does not make any leaps; neither does yoga.

(2–3) When the kundalini is sleeping it will be aroused by the grace of the guru. Then all the chakras and knots are pierced

and prana flows through the royal road of sushumna. The mind is released from its work and the yogi conquers death.

One thing is certain: kundalini is more than just a symbolic term for one of our known forces or faculties. It is a potential of which normally we know nothing, and one that does not seem to exist for the average man.

The chakras are occasionally perceptible in everyday life. In times of danger there is usually a convulsive contraction of the muladhara chakra; in the case of acute danger, it intestifies as the often-mentioned experience of "seeing the whole life flash through the mind." In sexual excitement the svadishthana chakra is noticeable. Best known is the influence of the manipura chakra on crying and laughter, which are related to the region of the diaphragm. One speaks of loving devotion as coming from the heart; it really involves the neighboring anahata chakra. The well-known choking sensation when a speaker is "blocked" relates to the vishuddha chakra. The index finger on the brow—"Eureka!"—means that the ajna chakra has spoken, and the halo on the image of a saint has its center in sahasrara chakra, to mention just a few minor characteristic signs of these unknown, yet so important centers in man.

(4) Sushumna, the great void; brahmarandra, the royal road, the burning ground; shambhavi, the middle way—all is one.

How easily one gets confused by big words. Certainly, this spiritual background is unfathomably profound. There are whole philosophical libraries on the "great void," shunyata, and a school of Buddhism is based on this term. Let us leave this sutra behind us as soon as possible, for nothing is more tempting than to delve into the depth of these terms, to compare them and search for their inner relationship. Yet how useless this is if one has not *experienced* the unity of all these differentiations in meditation. This alone is the way of wisdom, not philosophical brooding.

(5) The yogi should carefully practice the various mudras, in order to arouse the great goddess, ƙundalini, who in her sleep closes the mouth of the sushumna.

Mudra: the decisive theme of this chapter. A mudra awakens kundalini; it is set in motion through the practices we have learned in the first two parts of this work.

This arrangement testifies to great wisdom. What good would it do to activate this force without first having learned how to utilize it? He who wants to wake a giant first must test the sharpness of his weapons and make sure of his protection.

(6–9) Mahamudra, mahabandha, mahavedha, ƙhecari; uddiyana bandha, mula bandha, and jalandhara bandha; viparitaƙa rani, vajroli, and shaƙticalana; these are the ten mudras which conquer old age and death. —They have been given by Siva and confer the eight siddhis [on the yogi]. All the siddhas strive for them, but they are hard to attain, even for the Gods. They should be carefully ƙept secret, liƙe a box full of diamonds, and, liƙe an illicit relation with a married woman of noble birth, should not be mentioned to anyone.

(10–14) Press the anus with the left heel and extend the right leg; grasp the toes with your hand. Then practice jalandhara bandha and draw the breath through the sushumna. Thus the ƙundalini will stretch out, liƙe a snake that has been hit by a sticƙ. The two nadis die off thereby, because the prana leaves them. Then exhale—slowly, never fast. The sages call this maha-mudra. It destroys death and other sufferings. Because it has

been taught by the great siddhas it is called mahamudra, the great mudra, and also because of its surpassing importance.

Even the first practice in this new stage brings with it powerful experiences about which the text says nothing. So let us look at this practice a little more closely.

Once more we come upon jalandhara bandha. We have encountered it twice before (see Part II, 45 and 68). But we must not make comparisons, because the same practice can serve completely different purposes on different levels.

Here we must also mention the prerequisites for the above practice.

It is quite clear that the asanas of the first training period are taken for granted. Pranayama too is taken for granted, and is no longer mentioned. But for us there is something new.

The daily nadi purification must precede everything, in order to give the nadis the final polish, and then begins pranayama as described in Part Two. When the chest cavity is filled with prana (remember the bellows exercise) and the abdominal cavity is filled with apana (by means of the pranayama with protruding tongue), we can begin with this practice. Forget the outstretched leg for the time being. The head, lowered to the chest, presses down prana; through pressure of the heel on the anus apana is forced up, and by the pressure of the retracted abdominal muscles the two streams that have been led together are united into one whole, to an arch which extends from the two nostrils to the two nadis (ida and pingala), along the sides of the spinal column to its lower end where the two meet again at the mouth of the sushumna (which is still closed by the head of the kundalini serpent). But now everything should be drawn into the sushumna. And for this we go back to Part One, 28/29, and compare that exercise with the above. There as here, the body is bent deeply forward and thus places the opening of the sushumna into a favorable position. The sphincter muscle is not contracted, and the pressure on the throat is felt to be stronger than that exerted by the heel on the anus. Thus the now unified prana-apana stream is guided into the opening sushumna where it slowly rises like the mercury column in a thermometer. And this stream sweeps the kundalini along with it.

Now something important happens, as the text reveals: "The two nadis die off." In other words, the higher the prana rises in the sushumna, the less remains in the two nadis. In this third stage of training, the sushumna is not yet completely filled with the stream of prana, and thus the nadis are not completely empty, but some day this will happen. When it does, the yogi gives the impression of being dead. The body becomes cold and lifeless. Only the crown of the head (the upper end of the sushumna) is warm. Life and consciousness are contained solely in the sushumna, where life really originates. It is withdrawn from world and body. The yogi has become pure spirit—until he eventually exhales slowly and returns to his former state.

Can he really do that, exhale while physically in the state of death? We recall the second exercise with jalandhara bandha (Part Two, 68) where this state of consciousness was being trained. And now we understand the significance of that jalandhara variation, for here for the first time we encounter this strange state of "new consciousness."

(15) First he should practice with the left [foot drawn up], then with the right, until both sides are equally exercised.

(16) Now there is nothing that he should [prefer to] eat or avoid eating. All things regardless of their taste or even without taste are digested. Even poison becomes nectar to him.

(17) He who practices mahamudra overcomes consumption, leprosy, hemorrhoids, diseases of the spleen, digestive disturbances, etc.

This sloka is for the ignorant and curious.

(18) This is the description of mahamudra which confers siddhis. It should be kept secret and not given to just anyone.

And this sloka is for the initiated who knows.

But there is still a great deal more to observe and to do in order to reach the ideal state described, where the kundalini, carried by the prana-apana stream, rises through the sushumna. For instance, it is essential that the stream should not reverse its flow. The following practice will take care of this.

(19–24) Press the left ankle against the anus and place the right foot upon the left thigh. After inhalation, when the chin is pressed firmly against the chest, contract the anus muscle and concentrate on the sushumna. Having restrained the breath as long as possible, exhale slowly. This practice should be done first right, then left. Some say that jalandhara bandha should be avoided here and the tongue pressed firmly against the upper teeth. —Through this mahabandha, which bestows great siddhis, the upward flow of prana through the nadis (with the exception of sushumna) is prevented. Through this one becomes free from the snares of Yama the King [of Death], and attains the unification of the three nadis: ida, pingala, and sushumna. It also enables the mind to remain steadily concentrated [at the point] between the eyebrows.

This practice, as a rule, precedes the previous one. It is, so to speak, the overture to the whole. However, a third factor still has to be mentioned:

(25–30) Just as beauty and loveliness are of no avail to a woman without a husband, so also mahamudra and mahabandha are

useless without the third, mahavedha. —The yogi, sitting in the mahabandha posture, should draw in his breath with concentrated mind. Through jalandhara banda he prevents the escape of the prana upward or [apana] downward. —Supporting his body by the palms resting on the ground, the yogi should raise himself from the ground, and gently strike the ground with his buttocks several times. With this prana leaves the nadis [ida and pingala] and goes through the sushumna. —Thus is effected the union of ida, pingala and sushumna [moon, sun, and fire] which leads to immortality. —The body assumes a death-like aspect. —Then he should exhale. —This is mahavedha and bestows great siddhis when practiced. Wrinkles disappear and the gray hair of old age. Therefore it stands in high repute. These are the three mysterious [practices] that conquer death and old age, increase the gastric fire and confer the siddhis. They should be carefully kept secret.

The real purpose of this last practice is of a purely technical nature. For there is no natural connection between the three main nadis which run parallel into the muladhara chakra. Although they all end there, they do not join together. This condition has to be created artificially, and it is accomplished by this practice.

Now the preceding practice [mahabandha] can be carried out successfully, followed by the first one mentioned above [mahamudra]. Thus the three practices constitute one unit: the kundalini yoga constitutes both the high point of hatha yoga and a part of raja yoga.

(31) These are performed in eight different ways. Daily, every three hours. This creates good and eliminates evil. He who masters it has to practice this unusual procedure only moderately.

Both text and commentary are silent about the eight different ways of practice, for therein lies a secret teaching. The kundalini, as we know, rises from muladhara chakra through five further chakras to sahasrara chakra, so in all we have seven chakras. However, the seven stations are not simply traversed progressively one after the other, in the natural course of systematic practice. We run into some difficulties here, for each chakra is assigned a specific element:

1. Muladhara chakra: the element of *earth*
2. Svadhishthana chakra: the element of *water*
3. Manipura chakra: the element of *fire*
4. Anahata chakra: the element of *air*
5. Vishuddha chakra: the element of *ether*
6. Ajna chakra: the element of *consciousness*
7. Sahasrara chakra: the *divine* element.

These elements have nothing to do with what is known to us as the density of matter. Rather they are planes of vibrations as required for the creation of the respective forms of matter.

Now prana is, as we know, a life current, and a current consists of vibrations. The kundalini was aroused by the prana current, as soon as this reached the vibration level of muladhara chakra, that of the "earth elements." If the prana current is to traverse the other chakras it will accordingly have to be transformed or modulated seven times. If the yogi is unable to do this, he cannot reach the goal of raja yoga. And in order to realize this goal there are, as this sloka says, eight different ways of practice.[3]

3. Why are eight varieties of practice mentioned here when there are only seven? With this logical question we touch upon an area that will cause a great deal of discussion among Western yoga researchers, for it concerns the revelation of a secret that is still kept closely guarded: the

To be more specific: these are not methods of practice in the sense of the hatha yoga practices discussed so far. They are yantra meditations and mantra recitations.

To each chakra are attributed a visual and verbal symbol, which are transmitted orally to the student by his guru only after an initiation ceremony. Both are strictly secret, and are unattainable to the uninitiated. (The well-known chakra charts with the lotus leaves and the sound symbols are not identical with the secret yantras and mantras, although they derive much from them.)

The beginner naturally needs more time for each individual practice than the master does. So if he goes through these eight practices one by one every three hours, and if he needs an hour for each (as is usually the case for beginners), then he will need more than eight hours of practice daily; this is the least that is demanded from the beginner. Moving from chakra to chakra, a master of kundalini yoga completes all the stages with a single breath, which, however, may last for several hours. Due to the purity of his nadis, he now has the power to keep the prana in his body active as long as he likes, so that the feeling of shortness of breath does not arise. The gross organs have been put out of commission, and the few fine organs that are still active draw their oxygen supply through the pores.

This closes the description of the first decisive stages of raja yoga: the successful attempt to activate the kundalini. As stated, it is a stage that proves important, but is one that is still far from exhausting all the secret possibilities and the prerequisites for complete success. What follows is even stranger and, unfortunately, even more difficult to understand. Let's try.

---

teaching that the kundalini should be led *beyond* sahasrara chakra. Many passages in the Tantras and the Puranas point to this secret teaching in a veiled way. This will not be discussed further in this book, for in Hatha Yoga Pradipika there are, apart from this passage, no references to it.

CHAPTER 8

THE NECTAR

(32–37) When the tongue is bent back into the gullet and the eyes are fastened upon the point between the eyebrows, this is khecari mudra. When the membrane below the tongue is cut, and the tongue is shaken and milked, one can extend its length until it touches the eyebrows. Then khecari mudra is successful. —Take a clean, shining knife and cut the breadth of a hair into the fine membrane that connects the tongue with the lower part of the mouth [the froenum lignum]. Then rub that area with a mixture of salt and turmeric powder. After seven days again cut a hair's breadth. Follow this for six months. The membrane is then completely separated. When the yogi now curls his tongue upward and back he is able to close the place where the three paths meet. The bending back of the tongue is khecari mudra and [the closing of the three paths] is akasha chakra.

Here again some fundamental questions arise. The indignant objection of the reader, although at this point it represents a suspect prejudice, is quite understandable from a mortal point of view. But, as we know, a great deal of yoga is not accessible to the logical mind, and thus the "reasonable" average thinker will reject the more essential part of yoga because much of it (seen from his point of view) is nonsense. He will even be right, for a logical sense that satisfies the mind in a logical, materially purposeful manner, is lacking in the key points of yoga. It is non-sense for the scientific explorer and deep-sense for the experiencer.

The "three paths" are closed: the nasal passage, the pharynx, and the trachea. This is the *vas bene clausum* of the alchemists.

There are three ways to close the gates: with the natural muscles of the organs concerned; with the fingers; and from the inside, as taught here. To the logician it may all seem the same, whichever method is used. But let him test whether it really is all the same. Close your eyes and mouth and hold your breath. Nothing happens. Then close your ears with the thumbs, the eyes with the index fingers, the nostrils with the middle fingers, and the mouth with the remaining fingers. How the sensation with this type of closure differs from the first one is easily determined in this way. Now, in order to get some impression of the third method described above, have someone else close your passages according to the second set of instructions. And again the sensation will be different. This becomes especially impressive once the breath runs out. Suddenly you are at the mercy of another; you experience dependency, lack of freedom. On a small scale you experience the fear of death, this feeling of being helplessly at the mercy of death that actually means being handed over to one's own inadequacies.

(38) *The yogi who remains but half a minute in this position [with upturned tongue and imperturbable calm] is free from illness, old age and death.*

Try to imagine the feelings of a person in this situation. The tongue is far back in the throat; there is no breath. There is, however, a growing fear as to what may happen if one does not succeed in bringing the tongue back to normal. To have to remain for as little as half a minute in this terrible anxiety can lead to insanity. But as long as the danger of fear exists no guru will advocate this practice, for the dreaded will most assuredly happen the moment panic arises. Only with calm reflection can the tongue be brought back to its natural position, and the face of the yogi will tell the apprehensive spectator how difficult it is, and that it really is a matter of life or death. Yet he who is so unperturbed in the face of death that even this possibility cannot seriously disturb his equilibrium, has the means in his hand to pass consciously through the darkest regions of creation and dissolution. He is free from that which death represents to the average mortal: the final judgment that he must face in fetters.

(39) For him who masters this khecari mudra there will be no more [physical helplessness in bodily conditioned situations such as] illness, death, mental sluggishness, hunger, thirst, or cloudiness in thinking.

He is no longer subject to the overpowering law of nature, whose most painful aspect is the fact that all spiritual processes are sacrificed to this law. He remains undisturbed and calm even at the time of death, and thus deprives it of its dark power.

(40) He is free from [the laws of] karma and time has no power over him.

Fear in the state of helplessness is chiefly the panic-stricken thought: "What is going to happen?" It is uncertainty about the future, and thus involvement in time. But he for whom time does not exist is not troubled by its uncertainty. Karma, the Indian concept of fate based on the immutable law of causality, of cause and effect, is suspended when time does not exist. Only a *process,* i.e. a time-conditioned event, can cause a time-

112

conditioned effect. A *state*—a situation unconditioned by time (which we cannot comprehend, because thinking is a process, not a state)—is cause and effect in not as dynamic sequence but as static *ens*. Karma is the effect (dynamic) of the deed (active). The self-contained, meditative state that has freed itself from the time-space conditioned outside world is karmically neutral (static, passive). When time is conquered there is no more karma.

(41) The mudra is called khecari by the siddhas because the mind as well as the tongue remains in "ether" for the duration of the practice.[4]

Ether, a vibration plane in the universe, is finer than all that is composed of atoms and molecules, and thus is an intermediary between the world of atoms and the world of consciousness. Science has not as yet made a final decision concerning the existence or non-existence of ether, the *quinta essentia* of matter. But the yogi cannot waste his time with the changing fashion of science. While science investigates, he continues to build with his "unproven theories."

(42–43) Once he has closed the throat in khecari mudra he cannot be aroused by the most passionate embrace, and even if he were in the state of an ecstatic lover he still could negate the result through certain practices.[5]

The example of the most compelling temptation is presented here to prove that through khecari mudra the state of complete and

4. The commentary breaks down the word *khecari* into the root *kha* = the empty sphere of the sky, and the root *car* = to move. The real origin of *khecari* is *khecar* = sun. The reason for this we will see later.
5. These two slokas have been rather freely translated. The reason is given in Part Three, 84.

absolute absorption in meditation is possible. We know that one of the preparations of the yogis who allow themselves to be buried for days or weeks is khecari mudra. In this state all bodily functions are suspended for the time being, and the body appears to be dead, because the activating, life-giving prana is absorbed in the sushumna.

But it is not only prana that is isolated. What else? Is it really possible that the upturned tongue can produce such mysterious results?

(44) He who with upcurled tongue and concentrated mind drinks the nectar conquers death in 15 days—provided he masters yoga.

We recall the legend of the churning of the ocean of milk where from this ocean, with the aid of the world mountain, the nectar of life was to be produced. The mountain of the world, so we learned, is, in the human universe, the spinal column, the carrier of the life centers. The snake, wound around the mountain, is kundalini, the potential divine force of nature. The gods who pulled on one end symbolize the higher life forces; the demons on the other end represent sheer physical forces. The tortoise that supported the mountain is the power of yoga, of divine origin and universal.

But what is the ocean of milk, and what is the nectar? That is the theme of this chapter. We hear at the beginning that the kapha current of the life force is called nectar (soma). And where is the source of the current that is said to turn into poison if the student's balance is disturbed?

The cosmology of the "Puranas," the ancient Indian garland of legends (and a treasure trove of the secret teachings, if one knows how to read it) tells us that the ocean of milk lies between the Isles of Shaka and Pushkara (*Bhagavata Purana* V, 20). Shaka is the mythological name for ajna chakra, between the eyebrows, and Pushkara that of the sahasrara chakra at the crown of the head. Between these two centers lies the ocean of milk, the source of the nectar. That is where the kapha current originates.

This shows that kapha, the nectar, is not just any kind of secretion, for the primary functional and structural elements cannot be delineated so simply. True, the explanation that the inversion of the tongue diverts the kapha current, i.e. the biological process of evolution (or at least part of it) is not evident; we have to accept this as a given fact. Irregularities in the course of this current or process, which as a rule lead to illness, are produced at will and utilized for positive purposes. Through "supreme spirituality," a physical process is transmuted into a spiritual one.

No one can tell what this fluid is, if indeed it is a fluid. Is it a glandular secretion? Possibly. Most likely, yes. But this should not tempt us to make fruitless speculations. In any case, the tip of the upcurled tongue touches a point on the mucous membrane and through this touch some process of endocrine secretion is altered.

(45) The yogi who daily saturates his body with the nectar that flows from the "moon" is not harmed by poisons even when bitten by the snake Taskshaka.

You may think as you like about khecari mudra, you may consider the matter of the "nectar" naïve or ridiculous; the fact remains that there are countless yogis who can take even large quantities of deadly poisons without any harm to their bodies. This fact has been verified by medical authorities.

115

(46) Just as fire burns as long as there is wood, as the lamp burns as long as the oil and the wick last, so also the life germ [jivan] remains in the body while it is regulated by the "beams of the moon" [nectar].

The source of the nectar is the "moon" in the area of the brain stem. The "cooling beams of the moon," a term known in the mythologies of all countries, drip into the "fire of the sun" that burns in the region of the diaphragm and, so to speak, represents the flame of life (solar plexus). But the nectar is not fuel for this fire; to the contrary, it subdues and regulates the embers that are constantly being fanned into new life by the vata current. It is a direct, active messenger of consciousness to the functions of the vegetative system. When the supply is impeded we have fever; with an oversupply the fire becomes weak. When the demons of coarse bodily nature, while churning the ocean of milk, prematurely sampled the nectar before it had been wisely apportioned to them by the gods of mind, they poisoned themselves because the organic balance was disturbed.

(47–49) Daily he may "eat the flesh of the cow" and "drink wine," still he will remain a son of noble family. The word "cow" [go] means tongue. When one lets it penetrate into the throat it is called "to eat the flesh of the cow," and this destroys all sins. —When the tongue enters the throat there ensues great heat in the body. This causes the nectar to flow from "the moon," and that is what is called "drinking wine" [amara-varuni].*

*"In the above two stanzas is given an excellent instance of the way the Hindu occult writers veil their real meaning under apparently absurd symbols. The principle seems to be this. They thought that the very absurdity of the symbol and its inconsistency with the subject in hand would force the reader to think that there was something under it and so he should look deeper for an explanation of this absurdity. A misconception

116

In order to fan the fire of "burning asceticism" the nectar has to be diverted from its usual course into the fire of life. But the stream is not only diverted; it is also utilized in other ways.

(50–51) When it remains pressed in the throat passage, the tongue is able to receive the nectar "beams of the moon," which are [simultaneously] salty, hot, and pungent, but also like milk, honey, and ghee. Then all diseases are eliminated, and also old age. Thus he will be able to teach all the Vedas and the Shastras; and he has power to attract the damsels of the siddhas. —He who with upturned gaze and tongue in throat meditates on kundalini [parashakti] and drinks from the pure source of the nectar stream that flows from the "moon" in the head into the 16-petaled lotus [the vishuddha chakra], he will be free from all diseases and will live long with a beautiful body, delicate as a lotus petal—if during practice he keeps prana under control.

Here we have the answer to the question: "Where does the nectar flow once it is deviated from its natural course, the fire of life (solar plexus)?" The tongue guides it into the vishuddha chakra (in the throat), i.e. into the most important one, the 16-petaled lotus that carries the sound *a*, the primeval sound which even precedes *Om (Aum)*. Thus he is enabled to teach all the Vedas and the Shastras. Here we cannot help but think of the saying: "His words flow like nectar from his lips" —like a nectar that flows from his mind.

In vishuddha chakra (so the scriptures tell us) the birth of the word takes place. Cognition here becomes word.

---

of this rule seems to have given rise to many absurd interpretations of really occult symbols, and many pernicious practices that promote animal tendencies and passions. As examples of these . . . the whole mystic terminology of the Tantras that has given rise to so many disgusting practices." (Iyangar, *op. cit.*, p. 58 f.) —Trans.

The fruit from the Tree of Knowledge gets stuck in Adam's throat, and paradise is lost. The poison that the gods churn from the ocean of milk is swallowed by Siva, and it remains in his throat which becomes blue. The fruit gets stuck in Snow White's throat too—the undigested fruit of the dark mother aspect, which she does not recognize as her fruit and thus is unable to "digest."

The fruit of the process of evolution is always twofold: nectar for the perfect one, poison for the all-too-human one. The nectar is at the highest level, in its noblest aspect, pure spirit. For the materialist it is just what its gross aspect represents: the manifold bodily secretions. Just as the crude aspect of alcohol is merely a liquid—until it is imbibed. Then it shows its strength.

(52) Inside of the upper part of Mount Meru—that is the sushumna—there, in the opening, nectar is secreted. He who has a pure sattva mind, not overshadowed by rajas and tamas, therein recognizes the Truth [his own Atman]. It is the gully into which the currents discharge themselves. From the "moon" flows the nectar, the bodily essence, and hence the death of the mortals. Therefore one should practice the beneficial khecari mudra. Otherwise no siddhis will be attained.

(53) The sushumna, especially its [upper] opening, is the place of confluence of the five rivers and bestows divine knowledge. In the void of the opening which is freed from the influence of ignorance [avidya], sorrow, and delusions [of maya], the khecari mudra reaches perfection.

Just as breath (the vata element) has five currents (the five vayus), so also has the nectar of the kapha element, and so there are five fires that burn inside. However, the "asceticism of the five fires" (pancagni tapas) is a little different from that which is seen today at Rishikesh or Benares, where Siva sadhus light four great fires around themselves (the sun is considered to be the fifth) and try to slowly roast into the sainthood which is more distant from them than the sun.

(54) There is only one germ of evolution, and that is Om; there is only one mudra: khecari; only one duty: to become independent from everything; and only one spiritual state [avastha]: deep meditation [mano-mani].

CHAPTER 9

THE BANDHAS

BEFORE going any further let us recall one sentence: "Mahamudra, mahabandha, mahavedha, khecari; uddiyana bandha, mula bandha, and jalandhara bandha; viparitakarani, vajroli, and shakticalana; these are the ten mudras which conquer old age and death." So far we have learned only a few of these mudras:

Mahamudra: The joining of prana and apana.
Mahabandha: Preventing prana and apana from reverting their course.
Mahavedha: Connecting the three nadis by beating the buttocks on the floor.
Khecari mudra: Bending back the tongue.

The following three bandhas are not unknown to us, but they are discussed below from a new point of view.

(55–62) Uddiyana bandha [literally "to fly up," "to arise"] is so called by the yogis because thereby the prana flies up through the sushumna. Through this bandha the great bird "prana" constantly flies up through the sushumna; that is why it is called uddiyana banda. Drawing up the intestines above or below the navel [so that they touch the back and the diaphragm] is called uddiyana bandha. It is the lion who conquers the elephant,

death. —He who constantly practices uddiyana bandha as taught by his guru, and as it occurs in a natural way, becomes young though he may be old. —He should draw up the intestines below or above the navel, and within a month he will conquer death, without a doubt. Of all the bandhas uddiyana bandha is the most excellent. When it is mastered, liberation [mukti] follows naturally.

We have encountered this bandha twice before: first in the purification process of shatkarma. There it preceded the churning of the intestines (Part Two, 33/34). Then we met it in the next chapter when we had to raise the abdominal apana (Part Two, 45). In both cases the practice was mainly mechanical. Here, in the third case, it says: "because through this practice prana flows through the sushumna . . ." We now know considerably more than we did at the previous levels of training. There are more things happening internally, so that uddiyana bandha has indeed acquired a decisive meaning.

The inner process of this practice is as follows: In the two nadis, prana and apana have been united into one continuous flow, and neither a separation of the two nor a reversal of the current can occur after this point. From the nostrils to the muladhara chakra a current-bearing path now extends, or rather two paths, which unite at the lower end of the sushumna. From there the path again goes upward to the "moon." The flow of nectar is diverted by the upcurled tongue, so that the "sun" can now unfold its full fiery power.

There still remains one important question: to what end should the "sun" yield its strongest fire?

We know that the sun sits in the area of the fire chakra (manipura) below the heart chakra (anahata), within which dwells jivan, the germ of life. This jivan resembles the filament in the radio tube that sends out electrons as soon as it is warmed up. The "cathode rays" that the jivan sends out when heated by the sun are concentrated vital energy, and the practicing yogi needs a great deal of this for his kundalini. In order to bring this about the fire has to be led closer to the jivan, i.e. to the anahata chakra, and uddiyana bandha accomplishes just this. But fire cannot kindle without air, so the flame has a second task: to attract the prana-apana current by drawing it up through the sushumna.

(61–64) Press the scrotum with the heel, contract the anus, and force apana upward. This is mula bandha. Through contraction of the muladhara the normally downward flowing current of apana is guided upward. This is why the yogis call it mula [root] bandha. —Press the anus with the heel and press apana forcefully until it flows upward. Through mula bandha, prana and apana as well as nada and bindu unite to give perfection to the yogi. There is no doubt about this.

Through the pressure of the heel and the taut anus muscle the upward tendency is furthered and the current kept flowing. Here again, a practice that had little meaning for the beginner has taken on a decisive character.

We will get acquainted with nada and bindu at level IV.

(65) Through the union of prana and apana, secretions are considerably reduced. Through mula bandha a yogi, though old, becomes young.

Indeed, for the fire that tempers the life germ is fanned into new vigor by this practice.

(66–69) When apana rises upward and reaches the fire orbit, the flame becomes large and bright, fanned by apana. When apana

and the fire join with prana which by its nature is hot, then the fire of the body becomes especially bright and powerful. The kundalini feels the great heat thereby and awakens from its sleep like a snake that is hit by a stick, hisses and raises itself. Then it enters the opening [of sushumna]. Therefore the yogi should always practice mula bandha.

Should any nectar now flow into the fire, all efforts would have been in vain, for the organism would at once revert to "normal." Therefore we have to take precautionary measures which will support the work of the tongue, so that it only needs to intercept, but need not conduct.

(70–73) Contract the throat and press the chin against the breast. This is jalandhara bandha and destroys old age and death. It is called jalandhara bandha because it makes the nadis taut and stops the downward flow of the nectar which issues from the throat. When jalandhara bandha is accomplished and the throat contracted, not a single drop of nectar can fall into the fire of life and the breath does not take a wrong path. When the throat is firmly contracted, the two nadis are dead. Here in the throat sits the middle chakra, vishuddha. Here the 16 life centers are firmly bound.

We have also encountered before, this jalandhara bandha at a time when it did not have much significance; we are meeting it now for the fourth time. It will help if we follow the evolutionary stages in connection with this bandha through all four phases. In the first place it helped us to learn kumbhaka in pranayama (Part Two, 45). There it had only a supporting role. In the second case it suddenly had a strange result (Part Two, 68): it caused a state of mental absence. Though this was only to give the student the experience of such a state it nevertheless proved the overwhelming power of this bandha. Then it appeared in Part Three (10-14), where the first practical experiments were made with kundalini and the knowledge acquired thus far. The fire merely glowed and no harm could come of it, for the powerful key, khechari mudra, was missing. But now the fire flares up, and it has been brought closer to the life germ. Now all the supplementary practices, formerly so negligible, have a thousandfold greater effect.

The nadis have died off, so it says. Indeed, the prana-apana current now flows through the sushumna. The body appears to be dead, while deep inside an infinitely intense life is burning, more intense than any of the many known vital manifestations of life. If one touches the crown of the yogi's head in this state one can feel a little of it. While the body is ice-cold the center of his head burns as though in a raging fever.

(74–76) Practice uddiyana bandha by contracting the anus muscle; tighten the nadis ida and pingla [through jalandhara bandha] and cause the prana to flow [through the sushumna] to the upper part. In this way the breath is absorbed [it remains motionless in the sushumna] and old age, disease and death are conquered. The yogi masters these three outstanding bandhas, as practiced by the great siddhas [Matsyendra, Vashishtha, and others], and through which one acquires the siddhis described in the hatha yoga shastras.

The yogi now has the much-debated ability to put himself into a deathlike state, and to remain buried for days or weeks (to prove that he is not cheating). No one who has read the text so far will contend that this conscious death is now no longer a riddle. Even to the yogi who masters it, it is replete with mysteries.

Only one thing must be remembered: all this—that seems so

strange to us—is not essential. The yogi does not practice the ancient art of yoga in order to play dead, to remain for days or weeks under ground, or to squat in the midst of five flaring fires, on nail boards, or in a block of ice. If this were so we would be fools not to find something more worthy of our interest. Something is at stake that seems much less flamboyant than these imposing tricks: the perfection, not the distortion, of man; the development, not the abuse, of inner powers. This is a fact, and those who do not recognize it cannot change it, not even those in the homeland of yoga itself. Even in India it is hard to find a master. One encounters magicians everywhere, but the true master does not exhibit himself publicly.

Now there is a second method to divert the flow of the nectar.

(77–79) Every particle of nectar that flows from the ambrosial "moon" is [normally] swallowed up by the "sun." Thus the body grows old. [But] there is an excellent practice whereby the sun is deceived. But this we can learn only from the guru. No theoretical study even of a million shastras can elucidate it. It is viparitakarani, whereby the attributes of the "moon" and those of the "sun" are exchanged. The "sun" in the solar plexus and the "moon" above the palate exchange places. This must be learned from the guru.

On the surface, the practice itself seems comparatively simple, as we will see. The difficulties lie once again within us. But let the text lead us a little closer to the secret.

(80–82) In him who practices daily the gastric fire increases. Therefore the yogi should always have an ample supply of food on hand. If he restricts his food intake the fire will eat his body [instead]. —On the first day he should remain [only] a little while in the headstand, with legs in the air. This is viparitaka-

125

rani. Increase the practice time a little each day. After six months gray hair and wrinkles disappear. He who practices three hours a day conquers death.

Through a headstand, values are reversed. And what is so difficult about learning this?

First of all, we must know one thing: Among the asanas, the physical exercises treated in the first book, there is one that our text does not mention, although it is called the queen of asanas, and this is the headstand. This asana is called sirshasana.

As mentioned above, there is no great difficulty in this practice. And it is not the headstand that is referred to in the text as not being teachable through books or description. It is the process of deceiving the sun that can be learned from a guru only. How to exchange the position of the moon and the sun; that is what has to be learned from the guru, for this exchange is not accomplished by simply standing on our head.

But it does happen as soon as one has become accustomed to this position, as soon as the organism functions exactly as in the normal position. We know that through a radical change in consciousness organic processes can be influenced. Now we have to reach the point where consciousness does not register this inverted position as unusual. Then all the organs will adjust to it. How this is to be accomplished is the great problem discussed in this sloka. If it were a problem of meditation, it would be a comparatively simple matter for the experienced yogi. But if he does not want to fall down, he has to keep fully awake—and still convert his consciousness! This cannot be achieved through any kind of technique, but only through the suggestive influence of the guru.

This practice, by the way, is nowadays seldom encountered. Is it perhaps due to the fact that there are not any more gurus who have these suggestive powers?

126

(83) When someone, though leading a worldly life without observing the laws of yama and niyama, practices vajroli mudra he will become a vessel for siddhi powers.

The following slokas, 84–103, describe the vajroli, sahajoli and amaroli mudras. These are practices that aim at reversing the flow of the *semen virile in coito.* The purpose of such practices is clear: to enjoy all the benefits of yoga without sacrificing any of the worldly pleasures.

In leaving out these passages, we merely bypass the description of a few obscure and repugnant practices that are followed by only those yogis who lack the will power to reach their goal otherwise. In these 20 slokas, we encounter a yoga that has nothing but its name in common with the yoga of a Patanjali or a Ramakrishna.

Any technique that enables a yogi to sublimate his virility within his organism merits approval. Whatever he does outside his organism cannot be called yoga. For a yoga without yamas and niyamas does not exist. Even the very profound maithuna practices (i.e. ritual cohabitation) of the Shaktism cult can be acknowledged as a symbolic background of a religious ritual, but not this technique of uniting pleasure with the benefits of yoga. So let us take a detour around Orcus into the purer fields of kundalini.

CHAPTER 10

THE SHAKTI

EVERYTHING so far has really been only preparation. Everything essential has been accomplished, except the most essential: the raising of kundalini. To be sure, the yogi is now capable of going into deep meditation; he can put his body into a deathlike state; and he can fan or quench the inner fire. He has complete control over the functions of his body. All in all, he is master of hatha yoga.

But what of it? He is still only an insignificant apprentice of raja yoga. We have already seen that it is not the bodily functions and their control that count. Decisive is the degree of total perfection—physical, mental, and spiritual. Mastery of hatha yoga is only a preliminary to the mastery of raja yoga.

This final chapter of the third stage of training is concerned with the last, though the most magnificent of all physical phenomena: the guiding of the kundalini serpent through the various chakras to its highest goal, the sahasrara. Note, however, that it does not bring in the all-important phenomena that characterize absolute consciousness, the essence of raja yoga. The technical-dynamic process which is taught in the following will lead up to that goal to which Part Four is devoted.

(104) I now describe shakti calana kriya [literally: the action that loosens the inner power of nature]. Kutilangi, kundalini,

*bhujangi, shakti, ishvari, kundali, arundhati: all these are names
for the same shakti.*

Shakti is the name for all dynamic forces of nature. The release
of the shakti in man corresponds in its effect directly to the release of the latent shakti in the atom. Through nuclear fission
we do not call forth an external power, but simply release the
power latent in the atom. In man too repose unsuspected powers
that do not manifest materially but act with equal force on the
mental plane, which in turn reacts on the spiritual plane. We
need such an atomic spiritual power in order to reach the goal
of the yogi. With our threadbare everyday intellect we get
nowhere. It leads us, if anywhere, into a hopeless blind alley.

Where else can we find the needed forces for the highest
goal, if not from within our own selves? Since there is a path
to liberation, there also must exist the means to pursue it to the
end. And all the means that we require to reach our ultimate
goal, however high it may be, lie within us. The problem is
only how to release them.

*(105–110) As one opens the door with a key, so the yogi should
open the gate to liberation* [moksha] *with the kundalini. The
great goddess* [kundalini] *sleeps, closing with her mouth the
opening through which one can ascend to the brahmarandhra
(crown of the head), to that place where there is neither pain
nor suffering. The kundalini sleeps above the kanda* [where the
nadis converge]. *She gives liberation to the yogi and bondage
to the fool. He who knows kundalini knows yoga. —The
kundalini, it is said, is coiled like a serpent. He who can induce
her to move* [upward] *is liberated. There is no doubt about it.
—Between Ganga and Yamuna sits a young widow, arousing
compassion. One should despoil her, for this leads to the
supreme seat of Vishnu* [her spouse in sahasrara]. *The sacred*

129

Ganga is ida [nadi] and Yamuna is pingala [nadi]. Between ida and pingala sits the young widow kundalini.

(111) You should awaken the sleeping serpent by grasping its tail. The shakti, when aroused, moves upward.

Once more remember the churning of the ocean of milk. The demons seized the head of the snake, the gods took hold of the tail, and thus the work was accomplished.

Here we have the same process. The physically manifested powers, prana and apana, pull on the head; that is where the current flows into the sushumna, which is closed by the head of the serpent. The spiritual forces, however, work from the tail. We will presently learn about the nature of these spiritual forces.

(112) After inhaling through the right nostril perform kumbhaka according to the rules. Then manipulate the shakti for an hour and a half, both at sunrise and at sunset.

But didn't we learn before that we should practice eight hours a day? And now suddenly only at dawn and dusk! Here we have an example of how easily the words of a secret teaching can be misleading.

We have to understand that last sentence symbolically. The shakti should be manipulated for an hour and a half from two sides (head and tail), from the side of the sunrise (above) and from the side of the sunset (below). Here we must know the following: hatha yoga is comprised of jyoti (light) and mantra (sound). This passage means that the powers are awakened by means of the upper sphere of vibrations (light), which extends from the cosmic ether rays through the ultra colors to infrared, the rays of heat; and they are also awakened through the lower sphere of vibrations, from supersonic sound down to the lowest plane of vibrations. These are the means by which the kundalini should be manipulated "from the tail," the means used by the gods. The attributes that Krishna holds in his four hands symbolize these potentials. The symbol of prana is with Siva.

(113) The kanda [upon which the kundalini rests with its tail] lies above the anus and extends four inches. It is described as of round shape, and as though covered by a piece of soft white cloth.

In order to awaken the kundalini, the yogi has to know the plane of light (or color) vibrations as well as the plane of sound vibrations that correspond to the mulandhara chakra, and has to project the respective light and sound symbols onto that white cloth (of the kanda). But these two symbols are just as secret as those of the other chakras, and only the initiated can know them, for they are the keys to the most vital gate of yoga, to the spiritual atomic force that can bring blessings or destruction. Whatever has been revealed in the course of the centuries— carelessly noted and discovered by others, betrayed by talkative students—these secret symbols have escaped that fate. And even when single elements become known, the system has remained impervious because the initiated have always carefully kept the essentials to themselves. This is due to the extremely discriminating care of the teacher in selecting his students, and also to the fact that the spiritual results of this science mature only after the long and strenuous practice of meditation. If the uninitiated, even a scientist, discovered some of these things (particularly those concerning the mantra system), he would not know what to do with them. He is therefore skeptical from the very beginning; and it is highly doubtful that a skeptic would be willing to recite mantras that seem senseless to him

131

for three hours daily. Even the non-skeptic seldom possesses the strength to accomplish this from 3:00 to 6:00 A.M. Personal weakness is usually the best safeguard against the abuse of secret teachings.

Three components, when united, lead to success in guiding the kundalini upward: the spiritual, mental, and physical powers, as represented in the practice of asanas, prana, and light and sound meditation.

So once more body postures are included:

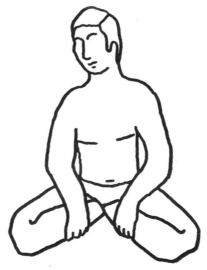

FIGURE 12

(114–116) Seated in the vajrasana posture (see Figure 12), firmly grasp the ankles and beat them lightly against the kanda. In the posture of vajrasana the yogi should induce the kundalini to move. Then he should do bhastrika kumbhaka. Thus the kundalini will be quickly awakened. Then he should contract the "sun" [through uddiyana bandha] and thus induce the kundalini to rise. Even though he may be in the jaws of death, the yogi has nothing to fear.

The earlier reference to light and sound actually belongs in Part Four, which is why the text referred to it only indirectly. Here in the last few slokas of Part Three, discussion is limited to the essentials of active yoga.

(117–122) When one moves the kundalini fearlessly for about an hour and a half, she is drawn upward a little through the sushumna. In this way she naturally leaves the opening of the sushumna free and is carried upward by the prana current. In this way one should daily move the kundalini. The yogi who does this is freed from disease. The yogi who moves the shakti gains the siddhis. Why talk about it so much? With ease he conquers time. That yogi only who leads the life of a celibate [brahmachari] and observes a moderate, healthful diet will reach perfection in the proper manipulation of the kundalini, within 45 days. Once the kundalini has been set into motion he should persistently practice bhastrika kumbhaka. He who is perfect in yamas and practices thus need never fear death [through his own kundalini].

The alert reader will have noticed that in these and the previous slokas only the motion of the kundalini is mentioned, and that she "rises slightly in the sushumna"—that is, so far as she does not encounter the resistance of the next vibration level.

We also note in the last sentence that when the kundalini is put into motion we should do bhastrika kumbhaka. How is this possible when everything stops during the deathlike state, including breath? The real meaning of the sloka is this: once we have succeeded in putting kundalini into motion we should emphasize bhastrika kumbhaka during the daily hatha yoga practice, because this increases prana production. The amount of prana available often makes the difference between life and death, for if the kundalini is led upward and (through some error in practice) the prana is prematurely exhausted, there is immediate danger of death for the yogi.

(123–125) What other ways are there to prevent the pollution of the 72,000 nadis? —The sushumna is straightened through asanas, pranayama and the mudras. —He who practices this with unflagging concentration obtains siddhi powers through shambhavi and the mudras.

The first sentence could be translated into modern language as follows: above all, do not allow the nadis to become impure, because then all else is in vain. The next sentence says: keep on practicing the first and second steps, for if the sushumna reverts to its old crooked shape the path of the kundalini is impeded. And the third sentence: in any event remain tirelessly concentrated.

(126–129) Without raja yoga there is no "earth"; without raja yoga no "night"; useless are all mudras without raja yoga. All pranayamas should be conducted with concentrated mind. The wise man does not permit his mind to wander during the [practice] time. Thus have the ten mudras been described by Lord Siva. One who is replete with yama [Part I, 17] reaches siddhis through each of the mudras. —He who teaches the secret of these mudras as transmitted from guru to guru, he is the real guru and can be called Ishvara in human form.

The "earth" is the activated muladhara chakra, "night" is the state in which the "light" shines bright, that light which we will presently discuss. From "earth" rises the kundalini, winding itself up on the Tree of Life to sahasrara, the crown of the head; and from her union with the highest principle originates the

134

fruit which she tenders to the seeker, the fruit from the Tree of Knowledge. Thus the yogi becomes Ishvara (God) in human form: *Eritis sicut deus, scientes bonum et malum* (Gen. 3.5).

Over and over again the concentrated mind is mentioned, the mind that must remain within itself. We have learned the art of the mudra. Now let's try to track down its secret.

(130) He who carefully follows the words of the guru, and attentively practices the mudras will obtain the siddhis, as well as the art of deceiving death.

And with this let us climb to the last and highest step of yoga.

PART FOUR

PASSIVE YOGA

CHAPTER 11

SAMADHI

IMAGINE that on the first morning after Easter vacation, a professor enters his classroom and announces: "Ladies and gentlemen, forget everything that you have learned so far. Everything that you have had to cram into your head so far was good and important, but it was only necessary for the lower classes. Now that you are working for your finals and are about to graduate, we will pay attention only to the essential, namely, the knowledge of ourselves."

Everyone freezes. All those years of worrying, the wakeful nights, the expensive books, the pain of memorizing—everything useless, senseless? The top student jumps up. He fights for the fruits of those painful years: his high grades which are about to be completely forgotten.

The professor smiles. "You are now going from the seminar room out into real life. There you won't be asked whether you have carefully analyzed Plato, but whether you can be a useful member of the State in the sense of the platonic *polis*. Hardly any of you will have occasion in his profession to work with tangents and pi's. Forget the rules and laws—but never forget that you have had the opportunity, through the laws of mathematics, to glimpse the great universal laws; and remember that these laws are valid even where we do not yet have formulas.

"Forget the sentences that you had to memorize; but remember that their meaning has now become second nature to you. It is in the forgetting of the mechanical process that the effect of real knowing is produced. Now the mind is completely free and can give full attention to its own self. If you still feel the need to have recourse to the first three stages, you are not ready for the fourth stage. You are ready only when all your spiritual efforts are devoted to this fourth stage. Once again, forget the teachings, for now you have experience. Let us begin:"

(1) Veneration to Siva, the guru who is in the form of nada, bindu and kala. He who is thus devoted reaches the maya-free state.

We have to pay careful attention here, for this devotional sentence harbors some vital information: Shiva who is in the form of nada, bindu and kala.

It is not difficult to understand this, provided one is willing to study the intricate symbolism of Indian tantra. However, that is not the purpose of this book. We want to turn directly to the practical side of the problem.

Let us imagine the strange case of a man who wants to re-create the universe. First he must decide what he requires. His answer to this is "quite simply" vibrations. What kind of vibrations would our presumptuous creator need?

Let us classify. The highest range of vibration is that of cosmic rays, which we term "light" for short; the middle range is "heat," and the lowest range "sound." But man too is part of the universe, and since every part of the creation is subject to the same laws, let our "creator" limit himself for the time being to the creation of man from his arsenal of vibrations. This man is a mechanism of the most manifold forces, and tendencies that in their *theoretical* totality bear the name of Siva. And since the composition of the universe is not different from that of man, and they both are subject to the same great law, this Siva is created out of the lower range of vibrations, "sound" (nada) and the highest, "light" (kala). (We will speak about the middle range later.)

But just as the universe is not a dynamo, neither is man a machine, for he understands "sound" as a concept, as a name, and "light" as image, as form. In this too he corresponds to the cosmos, where divine forces, finer than matter, rule in profound regions. But let us remain with man.

He comprehends. In other words, he not only exists but he knows himself. Everything in him is a process sustained by a force, a process that is in fact itself this force, the force of nature. And this force of nature (prakriti or shakti) is inseparable from him, the Siva. In fact, without this force he would not exist, for their relationship is the polarity of all beings.

Thus, as stated, man comprehends himself. And what he comprehends is not only the technical process of vibrations, but also the finer aspect of bindu, the principle of intelligence. Thus Siva is not only nada (sound) and kala (light) but also bindu (sense).

The middle range of vibrations (heat) is, as we already know, the metabolism. But this "fire" is not sheerly biological; it too has its finer aspect, its bindu. In Part Three, we saw how we can influence this fire in an indirect way by inhibiting it through the "nectar."

Now when the yogi wishes to produce his highest and lowest vibration fields to give new character to his personality (which consists of these two ranges of vibration), he would founder hopelessly if he addressed himself directly to his whole personality with all its fields of vibrations.

Instead, he has to learn to work on the "centers" of energy, the chakras. And his whole education is pointed in this direction.

What part do these chakras play on the different levels of

vibration? Let's analyze a word—something that has had a magical character from time immemorial—and let's try, with this word as an example, to clarify the inner processes.

Take your own name and pronounce it slowly, clearly, and audibly. A multiple reaction takes place:

1. The pronounced word evoked by the throat chakra rings out, But if you have carefully registered this sound with the physical ear, you have heard the *sound* and nothing more.
2. Now pay attention not to the sound, but to the sense. Not the succession of letters but the *name* is our chief interest. This involves the heart chakra. The word evokes a *feeling*, because this time you did not listen as attentively, but became more deeply involved internally.
3. Now don't pay attention at all; try to occupy your mind elsewhere, and let yourself be spoken to by your own name. Expect nothing, just be addressed unconsciously by your name. Again something else happens: you are startled. It is as though someone suddenly, unexpectedly, called you by name: something like an inaudible signal results every time. And this third plane of vibrations, the source of your personality, lies in the root chakra, the muladhara chakra, at the lowest end of the spinal column, seat of the kundalini. With this example we have presented the three levels on which vibrations, both light and sound, can manifest: coarse, fine, and abstract; or: perceptible through the senses, perceptible through feeling, and perceptible through intuition.

The corresponding manifestations of these three levels of reception are also threefold: physical perception through concentration (dharana), mental perception through meditation (dhyana), and spiritual perception in complete absorption (samadhi).

142

Before discussing these three methods of perception extensively in their relation to raja yoga, let us compare them with the above example of the name.

1. Noting with the senses (tone with ears or image with eyes).
2. Reception through feeling (What is the *meaning* of this or that symbol?)
3. Nothing; the reception "speaks for itself" because everything conceptual is eliminated.

Nothing much can be said about No. 1. It means perception and nothing more, in the way an animal perceives: pure sensory perception. This is the area of mechanical learning.

Processes on the second plane are considered more complicated, for here we have to presume an immanent spiritual primordial entity, which resembles a tuning fork in that when approached by a similar frequency of sound (or image) it will vibrate with it. Here the "meaning" penetrates the shell of appearances and hits the hidden opposite pole of consciousness, with which it condenses into a dynamic mental process. The fact that "meaning" here does not necessarily indicate the "logical meaning of the word" is intellectually difficult to grasp.

Before the student begins his meditation on the symbols suggested by his guru he has to root them and their inner meaning within himself, for it is not enough to adopt an apparently meaningless pattern of sound or form [mantra and yantra] and give them an arbitrary sense. He has to absorb the symbols so that they can freely unfold their natural forces to mobilize the archetypal spiritual powers, for such is their purpose. They must become as meaningful as one's proper name or one's own mirror image.

Before beginning to work with these symbols meditatively he must take his *mala* (rosary) and pronounce every syllable of

143

the given sound symbol (*mantra*) 100,000 times (*japa*) while viewing the corresponding form symbol (*yantra*). Once this is done—and he starts practice early [see Part One, chapter 17]—he has reached the beginning of his powers. By then the mantra has become name: the name of the deity that dwells within him. It is the name of Siva (or one of his powers), for every yogi knows "Sivoham," I am Siva.

Mantra becomes the key word, yantra the guidepost to the inner worlds whose source he must find. These inner spheres are fundamentally, primordially a dark, inextricable, labyrinth and even he who knows the ultimate goal needs a guide in order not to go hopelessly astray, for the intellect, like an unclean garment, is discarded at the entrance to this mysterious world. It would be of absolutely no help anyway. The symbol alone is Ariadne's thread, the magnet that pulls the seeker toward the other pole that is part of himself. In the light of everyday reason the symbol seems strange and incomprehensible, but in the depth of the unconscious it reaches a clarity that thought has never experienced. All this, of course, is valid only for one who has learned to delve below the surface of consciousness into the subconscious, for him who has mastered the art of meditation, the art of samadhi.

(2–7) I now will speak of samadhi, which conquers death and which leads to bliss and union with Brahman. —Raja yoga, samadhi, unmani, manomani, immortality, dissolution, emptiness-but-not-emptiness, the highest state, passivity of the intellect, non-dualism, beginninglessness, purity, liberation in this lifetime, the primordial state, and turiya (the Fourth State), all these are synonyms. —Just as a grain of salt dissolves in water and becomes one with it, so also in samadhi there occurs the union of mind with atman. Mind dissolves in breath and breath subsides. Both become one in samadhi. This state of equilibrium results

from the union of the jivatman and the paramatman. When mind thus is calm we are in samadhi.

The last two slokas contain three pairs of juxtaposed terms: mind and atman; mind and prana (breath); jivatman and paramatman. To understand the meaning of samadhi, we must understand the significance of these paired terms.

Mind and atman: "A thought [mind] has just come to me [atman]," says the student. "To whom?" asks the guru. "To whom came what, and where did it come from? Are these three separate things: you, your mind, and the thought process?"

Mind and breath: "Here is a process," the student thinks during pranayama, "and I am detached, watching the process." This reflection is the contrary of samadhi, the unification. Just as the theatergoer does not think: "Here I am and there is the play," but identifies with the play, forgets himself, forgets the process, is absorbed in the play, in the immediacy of a deep experience. As soon as he becomes aware of himself and knows he is here and the theater there, it is the intellect at work that destroys his involvement and with this he loses the essential, the spiritual experience.

Jivatman and paramatman: Jivatman is the individual self, paramatman the absolute, the divine Self. The universe consists of energy and matter, nothing more. This energy is always one and the same, regardless of how it manifests itself to our senses: as electricity, the motion of the air, the density of matter, or the beating of the heart. It is the energy that is inherent in prayer and the energy that answers prayer. The measure and the mass of this energy seems diverse only because of the various kinds of matter through which it manifests. Energy-in-itself is paramatman, "the energy which creates the personality of the living self."

If I now succeed in *experiencing* the inner meaning, the inter-

145

relationship of this threefold juxtaposition (sheer intellectual reflection is of little use), then samadhi (the establishment of oneness) is realized. The real One is then recognized.

(8–9) He who recognizes the true meaning of raja yoga can by the grace of the guru achieve realization, liberation, inner stead-fastness and the siddhis. Without the grace of the guru and without indifference to worldly things recognition of Truth, [attainment of] samadhi, is impossible.

The "grace of the guru" is his readiness to hand the student the key to success: the yantras, the mantras, and their application.

More important at this stage is the "indifference to worldly things." The professional theater critic is not supposed to be detached from the world, he must keep his intellect alert. Only when he no longer succeeds in this and is carried away by the action does he recognize and admit that what has happened to him is that which from time immemorial has been most important to man. There was a real experience; the soul was touched; worldly matters suddenly lost their attraction. What is really gripping is always the spiritual experience and never the intellectual, and the more neutral we become toward worldly (intellectual) things, the more open we become to real experience. The less critically we watch the magician's fingers, the more startling are his tricks. The critic may know more, but he experiences less.

Yet it would be an error to understand this uncritical attitude as blind acceptance of every deception. The critical intellect can absorb only the unessential part of a so-called truth, while real Truth reveals itself on a higher level, in the realm of the soul. Civilized man differs from primitive man in that, among other things, he separates and objectifies with critical intellect.

146

But with this he immediately closes the door to a real understanding of spiritual principles or religion.

Lack of thought is not advocated as a principle; the capacity to break the fetters of the intellect at the crucial moment is what really counts. Similarly, the ideal is not the blind fury of the raging elements, but the art to release those forces and then control them.

(10) When the kundalini has been raised through the practice of asanas, kumbhakas and mudras, then emptiness [sunya] *absorbs prana.*

Emptiness (from any discriminating intellect) and the process of the prana current become one; thus all inner forces are concentrated on the one process, the rising of the kundalini.

(11) The yogi who has raised the kundalini and has freed himself from all clinging karma will reach samadhi naturally.

(12) When prana flows through the sushumna and the mind is dissolved in emptiness [sunya] *then the perfect yogi destroys all karma.*

Thus Samadhi is the karma-free state. One could also say: the state of consciousness established in oneness neutralizes the effects of fate.

Indian religion assumes that the fate of man is the natural result of his deeds. "As you think and act, so you create your fate," is the saying. The less we control our thoughts, the more haphazard will be the course of our life. This is not a question of good and evil, but simply of doing or not doing, of a directing of our intentions and of their natural effect on our endeavors. This view is purely psychological and to be understood only as such. A divine power is at play only in so far as this logical law exists at all.

This karma (result of action) exists only as long as man is dependent on the relative values of this world. If his consciousness is established in the Absolute, independent of time and space, independent from all dynamics in static condition, then there is for him no action (not even a mental action or action of will) and no effect can take place, because effect only results from cause, and absolute, static Being cannot produce cause. Since karma is a time-conditioned concept, it is eliminated as soon as time no longer exists. For where there is no flow of time there can be no happenings, and when nothing happens there is no cause for an effect, and "cause-effect" is a synonym for karma.

(13) Salutation to Thee, oh Immortal One. Even time, into whose jaws falls the movable and immovable universe, has been conquered by Thee.

Samadhi is the most prodigious, the most far-reaching achievement of a yogi. For, being free from time, as he is in this state, he is also beyond the bonds of death, beyond rebirth, beyond all karmas, which hold in their clutches all the world's pain.

Of course he is not liberated with his first successful practice, for in this samadhi the karmic seeds that lie dormant within him are not destroyed. Each chakra controls certain karmic tendencies. Only when the kundalini force activates one chakra after another will the respective binding force be dissolved. For activating the chakras means gaining insight into the particular plane that has been reached. And gaining insight means dissolution of that specific karma. To mention just a few examples: In the muladhara chakra there is the karma of existence; in svadhisthana chakra that which is born from the I-Thou relationship; in manipura chakra the karma resulting from ambitions for power.

Samadhi, of course, is not the only way to liberation, but it is the most radical and within the framework of this particular yoga the most essential.

CHAPTER 12

MIND AND BREATH

MIND and prana, so it is said, are one, and thus mind and breath are interdependent. Where there is breath there is thought; without breath the activities of the mind will dry up.

These rather unusual assertions must be investigated further, for they are the core of raja yoga. It is not by accident that the German word *Atem* (breath), and the Sanskrit term *atman* (the self) have the same root. In our understanding, to cease breathing means to die. In yoga teaching it *may* mean death but does not necessarily. Certainly, consciousness in a general sense disappears along with breath, but what really happens after that we do not know. "Unconsciousness" is a meaningless term. Do we really know whether dying and being dead are the same thing, whether so-called unconsciousness does not encompass innumerable subconscious states? These are just a few problems relating to consciousness. We can become conscious only of events that reflect states, never of states. We are unable to grasp with our conscious mind a state that is not reflected by an event.

We are aware of some of our thought processes, among others those that bring the self into reality: this is "self-consciousness."

Everything that I perceive, recognize and judge is a part of my self, for my already existing relationship to the perceived indicates that the image of the object is already part of my store of experience, and that I therefore already have that karma-producing element (the previously-experienced object) "within" me. And my relation to the object is karmically conditioned, as well as karma-producing. It is thus an integral part of my personality.

To the Indian mind it means that we are under an illusion so long as we consider the self as a constant unit that which exists in itself and does not result from the sum total of consciousness factors. Thus the total of what I "know" (even subconsciously) is my self.

The illusion about human personality is fundamental. Where do we get our concept of human personality? As long as we do not get to the root of this question, we fall victim to illusion after illusion.

We watch our conversation partner, recognizing "in him" his personality. We consciously look above all at the eyes, presuming that these organs, designed for seeing, are also the mirror of the personality. But while we are thus watching the eyes in much the same way as we previously observed the sound of our name, they suddenly do not seem so important any more; in fact, they become insignificant in relationship to the whole personality. The same is true when we observe other single components: mouth, nose, cheeks, or forehead. Only the sum total of all makes up the personality. We realize that by observing the details we miss the essence. It is as though we were watching the glass rather than the image in the mirror. Then we realize that not even the sum total of all these details gives us the living image of the whole. But what is it?

The human personality *is* not "in-itself," it only *becomes,* within us. If we look mechanically at the surface we see nothing but the surface. Our inner being alone, not the eye, can see behind the surface. We have no specific name for this subtle

151

inner organ. Heart, intuition, feeling, soul, inner eye—all these are current expressions which are as familiar as they are vague, although they all express the right thing.

So let us look with nonmechanical eyes behind the surface, then we see the image of the object within ourselves inwardly. "Seeing" is only a small fraction of perceiving which essentially means to melt the (outer) image and the (interior) concept into one: simultaneously to see and to feel. And it is the same way with everything that we perceive with our sense organs. In reality it is not only sense perception, for all senses are only tools, organs of communication.

This, our personality-shaping inner world in its sum total, is atman. Yet the thousand little stones that make up a mosaic are, in their multitude, far from being a picture. Decisive is the manner in which they are put together into a pattern. It is this unity alone that creates the complete impression, not analytical observation; it is the inner perception that is based on something higher than the sum total of the individual pieces.

These countless elements of consciousness are united into the living total personality through prana, which has its source in breath. Thus the spirit, the human essence, is born of breath. And so, in a way, we breathe in the world, and breathe it out in the "form" of the personality thus created. The problem that concerns yoga is the creation of a harmonious relationship between the static personality components (the atman, the mosaic picture) and the dynamic personality (the creative artist's mind). In Indian terms, this means the harmonious marriage between static Purusha and dynamic Prakriti (shakti), between the human personality and its inherent forces.

(14) When the mind is still, united with the atman, and prana flows through the sushumna then [even the extraordinary]

amaroli, vajroli and sahajoli can be reached [that is, to volun-
tarily reverse the flow of semen].

In other words, there is no limit to the extent of accomplish-
ments.

(15) How can one reach perfection of knowledge [jnana] when
the breath is still living [in consciousness] and the mind [as a
manifesting force separate from it] has not died? He who can
cause prana and mind to become suspended, one through the
other, reaches liberation.

(16) Once he knows the secret, how to find the way to the
sushumna and how to induce the air to enter it, he should settle
down in a suitable place [and not rest] until [the kundalini has
reached] the crown of the head [brahmarandhra].

We already know why this is necessary. The chakras, these
activity centers of karma, have been penetrated, and since the
yogi's karma has thus been eliminated so that his mind is no
longer sullied and led astray by blindness and ignorance, this
illuminated mind can now melt with the atman into perfect
union. This takes place in the brahmarandhra, in the sahashrara
chakra.

(17) Sun and moon cause day and night. The sushumna [how-
ever] swallows time. This is a secret.

Here is an odd fact: if you observe the flow of breath for a
whole day you will observe that you breathe more intensely
at times through the right nostril and at other times through
the left; now the right nostril seems stopped up and now the

left. It seldom occurs that we breathe evenly through both nostrils. There is always a difference, no matter how slight. This is not due to a cold, but to the fact that the supply of breath through the one nostril has a different effect on the prana than that through the other. Breathing through the right nostril furthers extroversion; through the left, introversion. The breathing apparatus regulates itself automatically, so that through the lack of active elements the left nostril closes up slightly from the inside, causing the breath to flow chiefly through the right, and the active side of the body gets the greater supply. Mental fatigue is mostly preceded by a lengthy period of breathing through the left nostril.

One can (and frequently does) even out the imbalance by intensified one-sided pranayama. But the yogi has another method which, though applied externally, has an internal effect: He puts pressure on the side of the body which is overactive by lying on that side with arm strongly pressed to the body. Or he uses a special tool that he carries with him: a short crutch with a cross beam which he clamps into his armpit, while resting the lower end on the ground where he is sitting. After a few minutes the nostril of the side upon which pressure is being exerted will close up, and with this the field of prana changes over to the other side.

Normally the prana flow automatically changes in a regular rhythm, usually every two hours.

The reference here to the sun and the moon is not, as previously implied, to the source of nectar and its opposite pole in the area of the diaphragm, but to the ida nadi (moon) and the pingala nadi (sun). "Day" means prana supply to the pingala nadi (right nostril) and "night" prana to the ida nadi (left nostril). The cleansing of the nostrils (neti) which is part of the shatkarma (sixfold cleansing process) is designed to prevent an unnatural clogging that can block the natural breathing rhythm.

If prana is to enter sushumna then there must be neither "day" nor "night"; breath must flow precisely evenly through both nostrils. This in turn presupposes an exact balance of active and passive elements. In short, only he who has achieved complete inner equilibrium can have success in kundalini.

(18–23) There are 72,000 nadis in this cage [body]. Sushumna is the central nadi which contains the shabhavi shakti. This has the property of bestowing bliss upon the yogi. All others are then useless. —Guide the prana into the sushumna and kindle the gastric fire and awaken the kundalini. Only when prana flows through the sushumna will there be samadhi. All other methods are futile. When breath is suspended then [discursive] thinking also is suspended. He who has power over his mind can also control prana. [For] the two causes that activate the mind are prana [respiration] and the sources of karma [vasanas, latent tendencies]. Death of one [of these] is the death of the other. When mind is absorbed, breathing subsides: when prana is absorbed in the sushumna [not available to the body] then mind also is absorbed.

The deepest sense of this yoga will be understood only by one who is convinced that from physical process to psychological experience and religious phenomena there is one straight (if usually secret) path, and that none of the three can exist and function by itself. He who is prepared to familiarize himself with what naturally seems to be a strange terminology will find not only confirmation of the most modern knowledge, but the possibility of new insights as well, for the problem of relationship between the inner and outer worlds will always be a

155

topical one as long as the human race exists. The last word on it can never be expected, for each culture, even each phase of individual life presents new perspectives. It is by the great visionary works of antiquity that we are most deeply touched— we who have become so clever.

(24) Mind and prana are related to each other like milk and water. If the one dries up the other one also dries up. In whatever chakra the prana is concentrated mind becomes fixed, and where the mind is fixed prana is conquered.

The fact that men's cultural levels differ so greatly is not simply a problem of society; nor does it depend on ambition, or even on intelligence. It is really the chakras that cause stratification in culture.

Genius is the product of the highest development potential of that chakra by which it lives. As long as our mind is not nourished by that same chakra we only comprehend the lower levels. At the highest level our understanding is no longer limited. There we need no intellectual hints; we perceive the spirit everywhere, even in silence.

The chakra determines whatever level of development we are on, and this level determines the measure of our consciousness.

(25-27) The one is dependent on the other. They [mind and prana] *act in unison. Suspension of one causes suspension of the other. Without intervention the senses* [the indriyas] *become victorious. If they* [mind and prana] *are suspended there is liberation* [moksha]. *The nature of mind is like mercury: in ceaseless motion. When both are made motionless what on earth cannot be accomplished? Oh Parvati! Mercury is held fast and prana steady! Now all diseases are conquered and it is possible to rise into the air.*

Alchemy and magic—or only kindred symbols? Mercury is the symbolic square of the earth, the mulandhara chakra. The alchemical process represents the rising to the second chakra, svadhisthana. He who transcends the three lowest centers attains the fourth chakra, anahata, the vibration domain of the air. "He rises into the air." That is, he ultimately rises above the worldly spheres of earth, water and fire, into higher regions. As long as the spirit is not free from the lower spheres, it is not "held fast."

(28) When mind is held fast, prana is also held fast, as is the bindu in which the sattva element of the body is established.

In the first sloka of Part Four we translated the word *bindu* as "sense," (that is, the principle of intelligence). However, the word is so ambiguous that this translation is just a stopgap. Bindu may stand for: drop, period, zero, seed, the void. These appear to be quite different concepts, and one asks how the translator can add a sixth. Here we get a glimpse of the depth of the Sanskrit language, for each of these concepts has enormous significance.

Period (dot). It does not stand like a tombstone at the end of a Sanskrit sentence, but is the sign for vocal vivification. The dot above the consonant (which is always connected with a vowel) changes a dull *ka* into a rich *kam* or *kang,* a *ta* into *tam* or *tang, pa* into *pam,* and so on, through all the consonants. It adds vibration to the dull sound. It is especially significant that it raises *o* from the chest vibration to the *Om* sound in the head, the higher sphere. Thus it raises the physical sound to the chakra of consciousness, the ajna chakra between the eyebrows, and gives it meaning. In this way, the dot becomes the symbol for "sense."

The zero. Just as the dot is both a "nothing" and the symbol for sense, so is zero. By itself it is a symbol of no-thing. Added to a figure it increases its value tenfold. It gives the figure a value, a value that the figure by itself possesses only potentially. It catalyzes something essential without possessing a tangible value of its own.

The seed. Only when it falls upon fertile ground can it sprout. Like the dot, like the zero. And here the latent value is especially clear.

The void. Here again it is the meaning that makes emptiness purposeful.

> Thirty spokes unite around the nave.
> The void between them makes them useful as a wheel.
> We shape a pot from clay.
> Its usefulness depends upon the void that clay surrounds.
> The house is made of walls, windows and doors.
> The void between the walls makes it a habitation.
> We need what is;
> What-is-not makes it useful.
>
> Lao-tzu, *Tao Te Ching 11*

Now it should be clear why bindu means "sense." The sattva principle in which the "sense" is founded is fulfilled purity in the saint, who is all sattva.

(29–30) Dissolution [laya] *depends on nada. Laya produces prana. Prana is the lord of the mind* [mano]; *mind is the lord of the senses* [indriyas]. *When mind is absorbed in itself it is called mokṣha* [liberation]. *Call it this or that; when mind and prana are absorbed in each other the immeasurable joy of samadhi ensues.*

We enter a church and feel the sattva element that governs the lofty sacred room. Something like a shiver of enchantment penetrates us. It is bindu that (for a moment) transfigures us. We know that it has to do with the divine, to which this place is dedicated. We know it, but the inner concept of this "divine" is more than the word; it is that which speaks within us, nada. Let us recognize this: not the specific term "the divine" exercises its power, but the "inner something" that vibrates with this concept. Then the concept as such, with its thought content, dissolves (*laya*), and what remains is the experience of the spirit. This phrase, "experience of the spirit," already contains the duality: prana (experience) and spirit.

So much for our everyday experience. For the yogi approaching samadhi, the process is reversed: he has recognized the meaningful germ, bindu, within himself, and knows that the divine vibrations in him were merely released by the sattva element in the outside stimulation.

Therefore, like the ancient master mystics, he turns inward and finds liberation in detachment from the releasing element. For liberation means "nothing but" freedom from exterior influences.

CHAPTER 13

THE DISSOLUTION

On a cold winter night a wandering monk sought shelter in a desolate mountain temple. A cold wind was whistling through the paper walls and the frozen stranger huddled into a corner, shivering. He longed for a fire. Then he rose, for he had discovered the firewood he needed: the ancient gold lacquered wooden statue of the Buddha. He broke it into pieces, and soon bright flames were leaping up. With a cry of distress the guard rushed in. "Are you a demon, brother? What have you done!" The strange monk looked surprised. "What did I do?"

"You are burning the sacred image of our Lord! Can't you see? It is the Buddha you are burning!"

The monk smiled. "Do you believe we can burn our Lord? Don't you know that the spirit of enlightenment is indestructible? Wait until this mortal wood is burnt up, then we will search in the ashes for what is sacred."

The guardian shook his fists. "It will be too late. You will find nothing in the ashes." "Nothing?" exclaimed the stranger. "Tell me, did you hold sacred something that could so readily be destroyed by fire?"

The strange monk was Nanzen, one of the great patriarchs of Zen.

Everyone can test his relationship to the essence of a concept. Is it the thing itself that represents the value, or is it something subtler, something intangible? What is saintly in the saint? What is beautiful in the beautiful? It is our subjective thinking that creates values, and at times even eternal values. The thing itself is nothing but a clear mirror which will reflect that which we know within ourselves to be saintly or beautiful. This holds true not only for things from the outside world, but for our own thoughts and actions as well.

The activity of the mind always projects beyond our momentary situation, overlooks the essential, the Being, and focuses on Becoming. But it is only in Being that we can perceive the Absolute; Becoming is the relative. It is only when mind has become passive, dissolved in itself (i.e. separated from image and concept), unaffected by outside influences, that the Absolute presents itself in all as the true essence of things.

Will, however, is the great protagonist of passive contemplation. The more active elements the yogi can discard—breathing, thinking, desiring, acting—the more passive principles can manifest. And each passive element is a mirror of self-knowledge.

Not-doing in doing. Practice this
And know the unknowable.

Lao-tzu, *Tao Te Ching 63*

(31-33) The yogi who does not inhale or exhale and whose senses have become passive, whose mind does not register anything [no longer experiences subjective inclinations] has reached laya yoga [dissolution]. —When mental and physical activities have entirely ceased there results the indescribable state of laya yoga which only the yogi can experience. —When subjective views have been suspended avidya [ignorance], which is used to control the indriyas [senses], dissolves, and the power of cognition [jnanashakti] dissolves into Brahman [becomes one with the Absolute].

Avidya (ignorance) controls the senses. In other words, the attraction of the satisfying, purposeful, agreeable-seeming, influences the senses and in this way keeps captive the whole personality, which seems to have no higher means of cognition at its disposal.

To hear this fact and read about it will not cause any inner change; only when you yourself *recognize* it can you master the senses. Intellectual conviction, though well-intentioned, is only a sign of prejudice here, of pressure in the direction of a belief which can change nothing. And it is the change alone that counts. He who sees Truth is automatically changed. He who forces himself to change has only changed his opinions, but not himself.

This is the principle of the power of cognition: not to develop a new opinion, but to dissolve all dynamic active elements in Brahman. To contemplate and to be changed by that.

A man rising before sunrise searches for a lantern and cannot be persuaded by his friend that he does not need it. When he steps out of the house the sun rises, and he directly experiences the uselessness of the lantern. The thought of a lantern did not dissolve into another, better thought, but into direct process of realization, into "Brahman."

All opinions that do not result from direct experience are formed under the influence of relative experience. Experience is fate, experience is karma. "I have had this experience," says one opinion to another, one karma to another, one fate to another. In the light of knowledge there is nothing more to say, for man stands as living proof. The seed of karma lies in the stimulations of the outside world which can attract or repulse us. Under the influence of direct experience, a transformation occurs in which the senses lose their significance and sense experiences reveal themselves as conditioned and limited.

(34) Laya, laya, people say. But what is laya? —Laya is the state of forgetting [the subjectively colored images of] the objects of the senses, when the samskaras [impressions on consciousness, the seeds of karma] are no longer effective but are conquered.

But this cannot be accomplished by an act of will, for it is the acts of will themselves that block the way to evolution. There is only one way: to cognize and thereby know. As long as cognition is not spontaneous nothing really has happened and the process of dissolution has not taken place. Will always relates to the exterior, but dissolution takes place in the interior. So it is a question of letting the will die out, so that the clear picture of reality appears. Only in the vision of the inner image (which we cannot force) will relativity dissolve and cease to obstruct higher knowledge. True, our imagination is extensive, but never extensive enough to have a presentiment of things to come.

Only the suddenly rising sun which illumines the whole path ahead of us can show us not only the windings of the road that we read on the map, but all that which the best of maps cannot show: the grasses, bushes, stones, and grains of sand, the landscape of the true world in all its fabulous, infinite diversity. Are not all artificial means to stimulate presentiment ridiculous?

CHAPTER 14

THE SHAMBHAVI MUDRA
AND THE INNER LIGHT

(35) The Vedas, the Shastras and the Puranas are like prosti-
tutes [attainable to all]. The shambhavi mudra, however, is like
a chaste woman, carefully guarded.

Wisdom was never secret in the Orient. Secret are only the
paths to wisdom.

The intellectually created world of concepts has been dissolved.
Now let's return to the man who created a new world by the
two levels of vibration (light and sound), that interior world of
a higher life, which requires the stronger flame, the flame
which he learned to fan by khecari mudra. Dissolution is
samadhi; re-creation is shambhavi mudra, work with the sound
symbol (mantra) and the image symbol (yantra), the source of
inner light.

(36) Shambhavi mudra consists in fixing the mind inwardly
[on any one of the chakras], and fixing the eyes without blink-
ing on an external object. This mudra is kept secret by the
Vedas and Shastras.

What does the yogi do at this stage of training? How does he
practice?

He rises at 4:00 A.M., the hour of Brahma, cleans his breathing organs and sits down on his tiger skin.[6] After the introductory practices (such as the nadi purification) he venerates the three aspects of his sadhana (his personal deity): Keshava, Narayana, and Madhava as the three aspects of Vishnu; or Siva, Ganesh, and Bala as aspects of Siva. Then follows a complicated fivefold introductory ritual which leads him to his main practice, the shambhavi mudra. This takes the following course: First he speaks his mantra, clearly and audibly, in expression and intonation exactly as he has learned it from his guru, and retains the sound in his ear.

We will not analyze the sound in the ear here (see Chapter 15), but will concern ourselves merely with the question of what happens to this sound. The yogi must imagine that the sound is coming from one of the chakras. (The chakra varies according to his sadhana and his state of development.) And this sound is conceived of as so encompassing that it not only vibrates in the given chakra but is passed on—and this is the most important process—from chakra to chakra.

The mantra consists of various sound elements, each of which has a different function to fulfill. The introduction usually consists of the pranava *Om*, while the core, the shakti mantra, is a sound which influences the kundalini by its vibration structure. The framework of the mantra is tuned in part to the respective chakra; in part it contains other activating vibrations.

At the same time, if the yogi is not fully in possession of the yantra inwardly, he fastens his gaze upon the form symbol, the yantra, and imagines that this is the chakra concerned, the mantra that sounds within. For the deity, the chakra, the mantra, and the yantra, are one as name, image, projection, and

6. Only yogis who lead a strictly celibate life use tiger skin. The others use antelope skin. The reason for this is the difference in the power of the respective skins to isolate earth magnetism.

seat of the deity. The deity reposes in the chakra, the yantra is the expression of the divinity and of the chakra, the mantra synchronizes with the vibration level of the chakra, fashions the name of the deity, and is analogous to the yantra.

Add to this the proscribed color scale of the emanation of divine light and there is little room left for distracting thoughts. Many Indian and Tibetan texts which devote so much space to the description of the divine manifestations serve the yogi solely as means to reach the perfection of shambhavi mudra.

(37) It is rightfully called shambhavi mudra, when mind and prana are absorbed by the object, when the eyes become rigid in the contemplation of the object. Once this state has been reached by the grace of the guru [who gives the binding yantra as object], everything perceived becomes a manifestation of the great Shambu (Siva) and is thus beyond emptiness and not-emptiness.

Everything is Siva: everything is kala (light-waves, form, yantra, manifestation of the divine image in all its forms), nada (sound waves, sound, mantra, divine name in all its forms), and bindu (meaning, the divine, and the logos common to both the other spheres).

Before getting to the central point of this chapter we have to answer a question. The culminating point of Part Three was khecari mudra (the upcurled tongue) whereby the life process was intensified by the fanning of the inner fire, the middle plane of vibration. In what relation does the inner fire stand to shambhavi mudra?

(38) Shambhavi mudra and khecari mudra, although they differ in the position of the eyes and the point of concentration, are

one in that they bring about the state of bliss in the concen-
trated consciousness of the mind absorbed in atman.

The position of the eyes corresponds to the direction of concentration. In khecari mudra the point lies between the eyebrows
from where the nectar flows; in shambhavi mudra it is the
heart chakra, and therefore the eyes are directed that way, i.e.
to the tip of the nose. But this is not the essential difference,
although the real difference may be suggested by the direction
of the eyes. Decisive, rather, is the fact that khecari mudra activates the middle plane of vibrations, whereas in shambhavi
mudra the highest and the lowest planes are affected.

In the region of heat animal life manifests, while there is
little influence of the logos (bindu). However, in the region of
kala (the upper zone of vibration, light) and nada (the lower
zone, sound) there is present "the golden germ," bindu in its
plenitude. Thus the step from khecari mudra to shambhavi
mudra means a deepening of meditation and extension of possibilities.

Let us consider the form symbol in all its varied aspects: The
cross in Christianity, the half-moon in Islam, the star in Judaism.
The yantra has a *form* that we perceive and encompass with
our eyes; this is the coarse aspect. It also contains a "light" that
we perceive through our heart; this is the finer aspect, which we
will presently discuss; and finally the yantra contains a *sense*
(meaning, logos), the bindu, the point in which yantra, mantra,
chakra, and the divine unite.

This light, although it has its subtler aspect, should not be
considered mystical. It is first of all something that appears
quite naturally. The light that emanates from the cross has
more radiance for the Christian than for the Muslim, while the
light of the half-moon is considerably more radiant for the
Muslim than for the Christian. For these symbols have no radi-

ance in themselves. Radiance only unfolds in the heart of the devotee through his devotion, and even differs according to the intensity of the devotion.

The "inner light" does not imply an immanent meaning for the image symbol, but has a purely emotional value. It is not the meaning that is essential, but the kind of mood that it spontaneously induces.

(39–40) Direct your [inner] gaze upon "light" by slightly raising the eyebrows. Then perform shambhavi mudra as you have learned it. This induces samadhi. —Some confuse themselves by the alluring promises of the shastras and tantras, others by the Vedic karmas, and still others by logic. None of them recognizes the real value of this mudra, by the aid of which one can cross the ocean of existence.

One hazard which is more or less inherent in all religions is that they promise more to the devotee than he will be able to experience, unless he pursues his goal with extraordinary zeal. Because the Buddha did not make such exalted promises in regard to the divine, Buddhism has often been accused of being atheistic. But it is perhaps the greatest psycho-religious deed of the Buddha that, rather than promising bliss in the heavenly realms, he gave everything man needs to reach the goal of true religion, without obstructing the path with preconceived fantasies. God cannot be "spoken." He can only be experienced, and that is very different from anything projected through words. All too often a devotee is said to have "experienced God," when actually he has only seen the preconceived image of his own fantasy.

Mantra as divine name and yantra as divine form leave no room for fantasy. And thus these active forces of realization, to which even the physical sometimes submit, can be directed without hindrance on their way. For this path demands the whole man and does not permit any one force to deviate. Nobody has ever reached a high goal through dreaming alone.

(41) With half-closed eyes focused on the tip of the nose, the mind steadily fastened [on its object], and the active prana current of the ida and pingala nadis suspended [by guiding it into the sushumna], thus the yogi reaches the state of realization of Truth in the form of a radiating light which is the source of all things, and the highest objective to be reached. What higher state is there that he might expect?

"In the form of radiating light." Does this mean that the divine image here becomes the physically perceptible "radiating light"? Yes, indeed. Experienced mystics have testified that in their deepest concentration a radiating brilliant light appears before their eyes.[7] Here the same phenomena are evidently being described. What is happening?

It is not the object perceived through the senses that radiates, nor is it radiance from the heavenly spheres. A new organ of perception, so to speak, opens up through which the finer nature of the contemplated object is perceived. This organ has nothing to do with the senses. It lies in the heart chakra. It is so extremely subtle that the corporeality of the object is too coarse to be perceived by it, while it reacts directly to the finer nature, the light, which is directly susceptible to emotional values.

He who faces this stage of cognition uncritically without

7. Philo Judaeus: ". . . and the divine light precipitated itself like a flood upon the soul, and it is blinded by its radiance." Plotinus: "The vision flooded the seeker's eyes with light, but he sees nothing else, the light is the vision." Jakob Boehme: "Finally the gates of eternity opened; I penetrated to the inmost being and a wonderful light radiated in my soul. It was a light that did not at all fit the person that I have been."

recognizing its psycho-physical nature inevitably falls into the error of taking the luminous image as something self-existing. He believes that God has revealed himself to him in light, as it is often said, whereas he himself has only developed the capacity to recognize the divine omnipresence for the perception of which the average man has no developed organ. It is not that God has revealed himself to him, but that he has learned to cognize the Divine. A small but essential difference. The emotional value (light) of the Divine remains the same, but the devotee is now in a position to experience it directly.

At present everything connected with this subtle organ and the "light" is, as far as science is concerned, a matter of faith, just as the theory of the atom put forth by the Vaisheshika school of Indian philosophy was a question of faith until a few decades ago. The "revelation of the atom" was not a work of divine grace but of mathematics and of the electronic microscope; of refined observation. What was at that time divine in the atom still is today. And when some day the subtler organ in the heart chakra is recognized with the aid of a still subtler scientific tool, then the West will be more tolerant of the statements of yogis and mystics and possibly even surpass them. But the divine aspect will in no way be changed. Only one will perhaps accord it a place in the system of formulae, perhaps as zero, perhaps as bindu, perhaps as logos. Then one could also gain scientific knowledge from the Bible, for there it says: "In the beginning was the logos (bindu) . . . and the logos (bindu) was God" (John 1.1). "That was the true light that lighteth every man who cometh into the world" (John 1.9).

(42) Do not worship the lingam, neither by day nor by night. Only when day and night have been transcended should the lingam be worshipped—unceasingly.

170

This important sloka throws a significant light upon the whole of Hindu religiosity.

The lingam, the much disputed phallic symbol of the Sivaites, stands for this subtler aspect of all things, for the divine light; the primeval lingam consisted of fire. This is what is meant by the previous warning, not to mistake the radiant light for the manifestation of *the* God.

"Neither by day nor by night." We remember that ida and pingala stand for sun and moon, thus for day and night. Day and night are overcome as soon as the two prana currents are united in the sushumna, i.e. in samadhi. Only now is devotion real devotion and thus it says in the *Kularnava Tantra*: "Puja [devotion] lasts only as long as samadhi lasts."

Day and night are also the signs of time, which is conquered in samadhi. Everything that occurs in time belongs to worldly consciousness, to the image-forming, concept-bound way of thinking.

A worship that venerates the lingam as a concept is not the kind of devotion that is required for deep results, deep experience. The Indian does not make an image of his God for himself. This statement, which seems so paradoxical in view of the inexhaustible Hindu pantheon, actually finds its confirmation here. For all the images of deities are nothing but representations of various aspects of manifesting divine powers—with the exception of Brahman, who is unrepresentable.

Now some technical remarks:

(43–50) When prana flows naturally through the two nadis then there is no obstacle to khecari mudra. This is beyond doubt. —When the prana current enters the sushumna between ida and pingala then khecari mudra begins to become meaningful. —Between ida and pingala there is an unsupplied [i.e., with

171

prana] *space. It is there where the tongue performs khecari mudra. —The khechari mudra in which the nectar from the "moon" is collected stands in high esteem with Siva [who is kala, nada and bindu]. The incomparable, divine sushumna is blocked off by the inverted tongue. —The sushumna will also be closed when the prana current is suspended [by entering the sushumna]. This is the perfect khecari mudra that leads to samadhi [unmani, mindlessness]. —Between the eyebrows is the seat of Siva [of higher consciousness]. There conceptional thinking is absorbed. This state is samadhi [turiya] where death has no access. —One should practice khecari mudra until the state of samadhi [Yoga nidra, Yoga sleep] is achieved. He who succeeds in this will conquer death. —After mind has been freed from clinging [withdrawn from conceptualizing objects] it should not produce further thoughts. Then it resembles an empty pot surrounded and filled with space* [akasha, ether].

But what has happened to yantra and mantra? Why are we going back to Part Three?

Once the yogi has reached the fourth stage, he is all too apt to forget the technical requirements, which can lead him into the greatest difficulties. Again and again it must be emphasized: on the highest level of consciousness the inner fire must burn fiercely if the prana flow is not to cease (and with it the yogi's life). But the fire will only blaze when the flow of nectar is deviated, i.e. through khecari mudra. Thus once again high praise is bestowed on this mudra.

If no mention is made here of the shambhavi mudra, of mantras and yantras, we must not forget that these are inner events, while khecari mudra is a technical process. One cannot mix two fundamentally different concepts. Shambhavi mudra becomes significant only when khecari mudra has prepared the conditions for it and constantly renews them.

(51) When the outer breath ceases, the inner breath [prana pro-
duction] also ceases. Prana current and mind current become
passive when they reach their center of activity.

Human spirit is impelled only as long as it has a goal before its
eyes. Once the goal is reached, the spirit remains there for a
certain time. This period of abiding is usually the reason for
man's striving at all. An artist often searches for the conflict of
suffering in order to bring it into unity by resolving it in his
work. To be "desirelessly happy" is possible only when an
urgent desire is fulfilled, and relaxation thus induced—usually
the calm before the storm of new tensions.

When the mind of the yogi returns to its own Self after its
everyday sense-related activities it is relaxed, for with the sub-
siding breath during practice the active mind which lives from
prana subsides as well.

The prana he needs is in the sushumna and is kept active
there by the blazing flame of life. All life is concentrated there.

(52) When one thus practices control of breath day and night,
the prana becomes more passive in the course of time and mind
is naturally compelled to follow the same course.

For as soon as the prana becomes passive it unfolds its highest
effectiveness in the sushumna; and as soon as mind is passive the
real nature of the world of appearances is recognized.

(53) When the body is thus bathed in the nectar stream of the
moon it becomes strong and hardy.

In other words, when the fire is burning fiercely enough there
is no danger to life and limb.

173

(54) Place the mind in the shakti, [the manifesting power of nature, kundalini] and the shakti [as "light"] in the mind through meditation; then mind and shakti become one. Awaken the shakti by listening to the mind "with ear in heart" and thus strive for the highest goal of samadhi.

To listen "with ear in heart" is the most crucial factor in the whole process of meditation. This is the true insight, the prerequisite of all Eastern methods of spiritual training. Nothing else is of as such decisive importance from the first step to self-realization up to the arousing of kundalini, the inner light on the highest level.

(55-56) The I [atman] all in [empty] space, and empty the I (of conceptual being). When thus everything is empty [without time and space] then the [dynamic] intellect has subsided. [Thus the yogi is] empty within and without like an empty pot in space [akasha, ether], and also filled within and without like a pot in the ocean.

A pertinent simile! An empty pot at the bottom of the ocean. Water inside and out. Is the pot empty or full? Empty yet full; full yet empty. He who has inwardly understood this simile has comprehended the essence of raja yoga. For it is emptiness—though hard to grasp—which is the decisive factor in samadhi. But this is in no way a mortified spirit but a spirit that has been calmed. What this means, only he can understand whose mind has been completely absorbed in a great experience at least once.

(57-58) He should not think of external things; all personal thoughts he should give up also; abandon all subjective and objective thoughts. —The external universe [in its conceptual

diversity] *is a creation of our mind; so also is the world of imagination. When the idea has been abandoned that these projections of thought are permanent and mind is concentrated on that which is without change, oh Ram, eternal and certain peace has been reached.*

(59) Mind concentrated on the atman becomes one with it like camphor with the flame, like salt with the water of the ocean.

Then there is no I of which thought is aware, for I and thought have been absorbed into each other, because thinking is no longer attached to the object or concept but experiences purely the contemplative state. It is the absorbed observer of a great game in which it participates, and which is no longer a strange event to be analyzed and criticized.

(60) Mind and object of contemplation have been absorbed in each other so that there is no longer any duality.

The great symbol of this union is the union in love of man and woman. Therefore the Upanishads say: "The atman is as great as man and woman in close embrace." The bliss that ensues is neither I nor you, but the melting together of I and you in the mutual experience of the paramatman, the divine Self that is inherent in all that is created.

(61–64) The animate and the inanimate universe is a creation of the mind. In samadhi there is only oneness. When all sense perceptions are suspended there remains only the Absolute. —The great ancient seers experienced these various paths to samadhi, then taught them to others. —Salutations to the su-shumna, to the nectar-flow of the moon, to samadhi, and to [the great cit Shakti], *the power of absolute knowledge.*

CHAPTER 15

NADA, THE INNER SOUND

THE concept of prayer is well known. Here, however, we are not concerned with prayer but with mantra, though a certain relationship does exist between the two. Prayer is mostly expressed in the spontaneous, freely-chosen words of the devotee, while the mantra is bound not only in its sound but also in its intonation. In prayer the divinity is importuned; in mantra it is expressed. The prayer goes to the divinity; the mantra is an essential attribute of the divine, its "name." The prayer is a message bearer; the mantra is itself the message. The prayer is born in the mind; the mantra does not originate in the mind but it goes to the mind. Prayer contains the tendency that becomes clearly expressed in the mantra.

For example: every Christian prayer closes with an "Amen." "Amen" is in itself completely neutral until it is preceded by a prayer. In that case, "Amen" is the expression of all that the prayer implies. "Amen" is what makes a prayer a prayer; in fact it *is* the real prayer. The words that preceded it place it mentally and spiritually. "Amen" is the articulate power-potential of the divinity, the mantra. The mantra (in this example "Amen") is pure sattva principle. Everybody who enters a church, prays, participates in a ritual, or contemplates a sacred symbol experiences this sattva principle. Everything non-sattvic has a disturbing influence and is immediately conspicuous. Thus we go to church festively dressed so as to attract the full measure of sattvic vibrations.

Just as the inward light is kindled by the image symbol, so also through the sound symbol the inner sound is awakened, the nada, the most subtle aspect of the mantra, the sound in the "ear of the heart."

(65) I now shall describe the practice of nada, as has been proclaimed by Gorakshanath, and as it is accepted even by those who are unable to realize Truth because they have not studied the shastras.

It is "the dissolution of image and concept" (laya) in a spontaneous experience which has from time immemorial been considered the highest spiritual process. It is also the goal of the highest yoga, and all paths of yoga culminate in laya.

(66) Lord Siva has shown innumerable paths to laya, but it seems to me that the practice of nada is the best of them all.

The reason for this is perhaps the fact that it seems easier to deal with the sound symbol than with the image, and that the inner sound is easier to produce than the inward light.

The time has now come for the yogi to practice daily:

(67) He seats himself in siddhasana and assumes shambhavi mudra, listening to the inner sound that rings in his right ear.

And why not in the left ear? *Dakshina* means "right" but also "good, propitious, capable." So it really says here "in the true ear," and this is the "ear of the heart."

(68) Close ears, nose, mouth, and eyes, then you will distinctly hear a clear sound in the sushumna, which has been purified by pranayama.

The reader will perhaps feel impelled to make an experiment and to listen inwardly. Futile effort! He will hear nothing like this "sound." Why?

Would the yogi be compelled to go through three stages of hard practice if he only needs to close up his ears in order to perceive the inner sound? Are our nadis pure, is the flame, the source of higher life, ablaze? Is the symbol of the divine rooted in our being? Do we fulfill even the minimal requisites of deep religious devotion? Answer these questions before trying to listen to that which has from time immemorial been the mystic's most profound experience of God.

(69) All yoga practices contain four stages: introduction [arambha], transition [ghata], attainment [paricaya], and perfection [nishpatti].

This is valid for yoga in general, for the individual systems as shown by the division of our text, as well as for each specific practice; in fact for all things in life. There is great psychological insight in this sentence. May we learn that the third step, the attainment, is not the last.

(70–71) In the first stage [arambhavastha], when the heart chakra [brahma granthi] is pierced, we hear tinkling sounds like jewels in the space of the heart in the center of the body. As soon as these sounds become audible in the [interior] void, the yogi becomes god-like, radiant, healthy and fragrant. His heart becomes the void.

The sound which in the region of the throat was still sound, has now penetrated to the heart and there meets prana. A feeling rises like a deep happy breath and fills the heart, and the inner sound of the mantra falls like a golden dewdrop on this budding happiness. Everything that was beneficial on the technical path of the asanas is achieved in one moment of real experience, for:

(72) In the second stage prana and nada become one, and [this one] enter[s] the middle [heart] chakra. The asanas become effective now and divine wisdom arises.

Union is accomplished and the chalice with its golden pearl— that pearl which will later expand into a whole new world— extends upward toward higher spheres. What does it mean to grow upward? Why should we raise a lower sphere rather than simply go from the lower sphere into the higher?

We remember that the inner sound of the mantra is to emanate from one of the chakras. The sound then takes on the vibration frequency of the respective chakra; it becomes the principle that the chakra represents.

In order not to underestimate the value of this practice, we must remember an earlier practice that related to the physical aspect of sound, the audible sound in bhramari kumbhaka. (Part Two, 67) After the nadis were purified, the sound of a humming bee was produced. This happened, and the sound grew to a rumbling roar that made the world tremble. It was one of the first great experiences of hatha yoga.

At that time we knew no more than what we heard. Now, this impressive sound, created with the aid of the personal mantra, is not projected into space, but directed inward to a chakra; and this is our present situation.

(73) When the vishnu granthi in the throat is pierced [by the vibrations] it is a sign that divine bliss [brahma ananda] will

179

follow. In the sound box of the throat chakra [ati shunyata]
there a complex sound arises, like that of a big drum.

This is the subtler aspect of the rumbling and roaring that we
came to know in the bhramari kumbhaka, the effect of which
is here even more impressive.

(74) On the third stage a sound like that of a mardala [a dif-
ferent kind of drum] is perceived, in the space between the
eyebrows. With this the vibrations enter into the great void
[maha shunyata, i.e. sushumna], the seat of all the siddhis.

This too we have encountered in its gross physical form in the
bhramari kumbhaka, but since now the sound is not produced
by the vocal cords it is purely mental and that means more
profound. It is not easy to find an example of this in our arsenal
of religious experience, as a certain inner devotion and prayer
are prerequisites. Still even the sober modern man will be no
stranger to experiences under the spell of music.

"Arise!" the angel calls out to Mohammed in the desert, and
the sound symbol of the warning angel's voice is the sound of
bells, and thus prayer, or, on a higher level, revelation, becomes
passionate joy. The prescient sound of bells is the preliminary
to the revelation of the angel; prayer is the ecstatic revelation.
Prayer lives in the heart chakra, revelation in the throat chakra.

(75) Having overcome the blissful state of the mind he experi-
ences the happiness that arises from cognition of the atman.
Then he is delivered of all faults, pains, old age, disease, hunger,
and tiredness.

Greater than happiness is equanimity. Happiness is the goal of
man, equanimity is the divine goal. Immutable are the gods

alone. Humanity swings like a pendulum between desire for happiness and enjoyment of happiness. He who voluntarily renounces his happiness and nevertheless remains happy can no longer be measured by human standards (although not always by divine ones either).

(76) After the vibration has pierced the last knot [the agna chakra], *the forehead's center* [*of consciousness*], *it rises to the divine place. With this the fourth stage sets in, where one hears the sound of the flute and the vina.*

Let us stop analyzing. Our experience does not suffice to understand the meaning of the sound of the flute of Krishna, or the vina of the divine messenger, Narada. Those who have experienced this high state have become teachers from whose lips flowed the Vedas, the Eddas, the Avestas, the Sermon of the Mount, the Koran. The sounds now grow ever more subtle, yet more powerful. They are sounds that proclaim the Eternal Wisdom of God, the power of Ultimate Truth undisturbed and unimpeded by the word. Nothing is understood, everything known. The gates of the Kingdom of Heaven fly open, the eternal light is manifest, the music of the spheres rings out.

(77–83) When the mind becomes unified, this is raja yoga. The yogi, now master of creation and destruction, becomes one with God. —Whether or not you call it liberation, here is eternal bliss. The bliss of dissolution [*laya*] *is obtained only through raja yoga. —There are many who are merely hatha yogins, without the knowledge of raja yoga. They are simple practicers who will never reap the* [*real*] *fruits of their efforts. —I believe that concentration on the space between the eyebrows is the best way to reach samadhi in a short time. For those of small intellect this is the easiest means to attain to raja yoga.*

The state of dissolution [laya] arising from the [inner sound] nada creates this spontaneous experience. —[All] yogis who have reached the state of samadhi through this concentration on nada have experienced a bliss in their hearts that surpasses all description and can be known only by a god. —The silent ascetic, having closed his ears, listens [attentively] to the sound in his heart until he attains the state of oneness with all [samadhi]. —The power of inner sound gradually surpasses the external sounds. Thus the yogi can overcome the weakness of the mind and reach his goal in 15 days.

The power of the internal sound, its meaning as an audible designation of our personality, is a thousand times stronger than the logical combination of the sounds of letters which has really no meaning at all. The pronouncing of the name-word is purely inner sound.

Now the mantra is that name which is the common property of both the jivatman and the paramatman (the self and the Self).

At first it is separateness that impinges upon our ears. There is still an I and a Thou, the one who perceives and the one who is perceived: the dynamic mind is active. In the inner sense, however, all separative tendencies, all sound-conditioned differentiations cease according to the degree of their inner refinement, i.e. the degree to which they sink and become one with the static mind. The mantra becomes the true name.

At the beginning of an acquaintance a name only tells us *who* the person is. Later on it stands for the sum total of *what* the person is, what we have experienced with that person. The name then does not merely speak of the "Thou," but equally of the "I" and its relationship to "Thou."

(84–85) During the initial stage of practice various strong sounds are audible, but as progress is made they become more and more

refined. —At first they sound like the roaring of the ocean or like thunder, like kettle drums, or trumpets. Then they become more and more subtle until they sound like flutes and harps, like the humming of bees. In this way one hears them in the center of the body.

In Bhramari kumbhaka the yogi's ears may ring. In shambhavi mudra his physical ears are deaf, but the ear in the heart hears the fortissimo of inner prayer.
  So Lao-tzu says:

> The multiple colors blind the eyes
> The multiple sounds deafen the ear
> . . . .
> Therefore the sage cultivates his person
> And does not crave to see.
>
> *Tao Te Ching, 12*

(87–89) Even as the loud sounds [still] ring out, one should concentrate on the subtle sound [in the heart]. —One may well let the attention swing between these two sounds, but the mind should never be allowed to wander to external objects. —The attention turns naturally to the sound that has the strongest attraction.

Do not become impatient! If you are again and again captivated by the roaring sound in the physical ear then the watchword is practice and wait. Maturation brings perfection. Tone is outside, the ringing sound is inward. The tone releases the ringing sound, and that sound is fuller and purer than any that the ear can absorb. Consciousness directs itself to where it can expect the ripest fruits. No need here for thought. Who would ever comprehend music with the intellect?
  The mind resembles the bee, for:

(90) Just as the bee who drinks the flower's honey is not concerned with its scent, so also the mind, when absorbed in sound, does not care about the pleasure-bound senses.

The scent attracts the bee who forgets it while sucking the honey. The senses attract consciousness which, in nada, the experience beyond the senses, forgets them.

(91–92) The sharp iron prong of nada can effectively curb the [elephant] mind when it wants to gambol in the pleasure garden of the sense-objects. —When the mind has been divested of its fickle nature and has been fettered by the ropes of the inner sound, then it reaches the highest state of concentration and remains still, like a bird that has lost its wings.

(93) He who wishes to reach the mastery of yoga should renounce all his [restless] thoughts and practice with carefully concentrated mind the dissolution [of the world of senses] in nada laya.

In a concert, in the cathedral or in the poet's word, the "sound" is always there where an immortal spirit has dipped into the deepest sources of life.

(94) The inner sound [the bindu] is like a trap to capture the gazelle [the mind]; like a hunter, it kills the animal [conceptual thought].

Every word of every language has this inner sound. We hear it readily in the words of our own language which are to us more than sheer letter formations. But when we want to learn a foreign language—and the mantra in a sense belongs to a foreign language—then we have to start with the audible sound until one fine day the inner sound of the new words manifests itself. Conceptual thought then becomes superfluous. As long as one has to think about a foreign word, the inner sound is missing. We have adopted many "foreign words" whose inner sounds we have learned to hear and that have a meaning for us that cannot be expressed in our own language. The Japanese word "harakiri" tells us more than the word "suicide," the Chinese word "kowtow" more than the words "to bow." These are not words that stand *for* something; they have become identical with clearly defined concepts.

(95–96) The inner sound is like a bolt on the stable door that keeps the horse [conceptual thinking] from roaming about. Therefore the yogi should daily practice concentration on this nada. —Mercury distilled with sulphur becomes solid and divested of its active nature. It becomes capable of rising into the air. Similarly, the mind is made steady by the influence of nada and becomes united with the all-pervading Brahman.

Brahman is Om (Aum), and this is kala, nada, and bindu; Siva is the aspect of Brahman as destroyer, He who destroys concepts and liberates the Absolute. Siva, the dark aspect of Brahman, appears terrifying only to those who are afraid they will lose the world of concept, not suspecting that beyond this world there is eternity.

(97) When the mind [free of concepts] comes to know, it does not run toward the ringing sound [in the physical ear] like a [curious] serpent.

This is the famous characteristic of the wise man: lack of curiosity, because he experiences greater things within himself. Only he who is not self-sufficient seeks fulfillment in things. He who is inwardly poor seeks wealth in the relative world.*

(98–99) The fire that burns a piece of wood dies out when the wood has been consumed. So also the mind when it remains concentrated on nadam (and does not search for new fuel) gets absorbed in it. —When the fourfold mind (antakharana) has been attracted by the sound of bells etc., like a gazelle, a skillful archer can hit it with his arrow.

The Upanishad says: "Prana is the bow, atman the arrow, Brahman the target. He who carefully aims at the target becomes one with it." Atman and Brahman become one.

(100–102) The absolute consciousness [caitanya] cognizes the nada-sound in the heart while the antakharana [mind] becomes one with caitanya. When this has happened in samadhi [para-vairagya] all modifications dissolve and become abstract thought. This is the pure atman, free from all external adjuncts [upadhis]. —Space [akasha] exists only as long as the sound is heard [by the physical ear]. In soundlessness atman and Brahman are one [paramatman]. Whatever is manifested as sound [in the heart or in the ear] is a power of nature [shakti]. The state of dissolution [laya] of conceptual thought is beyond all form. It is divine [paramesvara].

As we have now ascertained, there is no real difference between the "inner light" (kala) as described in the previous chapter and the inner sound (nada) because in essence they are united by

*This is the only case where Rieker's translation deviates from the literal translation of the text, which reads: "The mind is like a serpent; forgetting all its unsteadiness by hearing the nada, it does not run away anywhere" (Pancham Sinh, *op. cit.,* p. 164). —Trans.

bindu, the sense. All three powers (kala, nada and bindu) in absolute form are Siva; in their active power they are shakti. Siva and Shakti are one as the inseparable cosmic lovers: energy and matter are one as source of the world.

Our imaginary human creator now has everything that he needs: energy and matter in all their aspects. The gross material aspect as sound and light; the subtle aspect as inner sound and inner radiance; the causal aspect as the divine experience of samadhi where there is no longer any difference between the three realms, where they once more are what they have eternally been: Siva, the aspect of dissolution of Brahaman.

(103) All hatha yoga practices serve only for the attainment of raja yoga. He who is accomplished in raja yoga overcomes death.

To "overcome death" does not mean to become immortal, for what is the body? It means power over all that which escapes consciousness at the time of death. Samadhi is more closely related to death than sleep. He who has reached the inner vision of samadhi will meet death with clear understanding of what awaits him. He has control over the state after death and the way to rebirth.

(104–114) Mind is the seed, pranayama the soil, dispassion [vairagya] *the water. Out of these three grows the tree that fulfills all wishes. —Through assiduous practice of concentration on nada, all sins are destroyed, and mind and prana become dissolved in absolute consciousness* [niranjana, the absolutely spotless, devoid of all gunas]. *—During samadhi* [unmani avastha, the mindless state] *the* [material] *body becomes like a log. The sound of the conch and of the big drum pass by his* [physical] *ear* [for the ear in his heart is tuned to subtler

sounds]. —*The yogi is free from all states* [avasthas, conditioned states], *from all thoughts. He is like one dead.* —*And yet he is master of death, of his fate, and his enemies. His senses have died away; he knows not himself or others. He is one who is liberated in this lifetime* [jivanmukta], *when his mind is neither awake nor asleep, and when he is free from remembering and forgetting. He does not live, and yet he is not dead.* —*He is impervious to heat and cold, to pain and bliss, to honor and insult.* —*He seems to be sleeping, and yet he is awake. Inhalation and exhalation have subsided.* [He is in jagra avastha.] —*Weapons cannot harm him* [i.e., *his now manifest real being*], *no human power can overcome him. He is beyond curses* [through mantra] *and charms* [yantra]. —*But as long as prana does not enter the sushumna and reach its highest goal at the crown of the head* [the bramaradhra], *as long as the absolute is not manifested in samadhi,* [as long as the bindu does not come under control by restraint of breath,] *as long as the I does not become one with the It, so long are those who talk about dissolution in Brahman mere babblers and prevaricators.*

EPILOGUE

When I review what I could gather from the few hidden saints I met in India my impression is twofold. The state of enlightenment, the state that precedes sainthood, is positively the greatest and most desirable goal of all. One still is a human being, but no longer a victim of nature; natural laws still prevail, but impose no burdens. One still has needs, but is not dependent on them. One feels and acts, but one does not act due to feelings; the aim is always to be in tune with cosmic harmony rather than to give satisfaction to the ego. The Truth of absolute harmony which includes the creatures and the Creator: that is the sign of enlightenment, absolute humanness. But the saint of the last stage is beyond everything human. He is a single sound that does not blend into a harmony of any kind, for he already occupies a higher plane of existence, one through which the enlightened one passes only at the time of death, or rather after death, when his individuality is dissolved. A man who begins to outgrow worldly conditions will be reborn into the level of existence he has reached. The saint of the highest stage passes through this condition in his inner consciousness before his earthly death, because he has succeeded in freeing himself from everything that binds others to the world. Again and again I had the impression, and saw it confirmed from many sides, that the enlightened one represents the most perfect human being, while the saint on the highest level could in many respects no longer be measured by human standards: obvious omniscience paired with the symptoms of insanity, but nevertheless with the distinguishing signs of a genius. Phenomenal manifestations such as complete renunciation of sleep and food; suspension of all natural functions such as growth of hair on the head, perspiration, elimination; complete absence of signs of age, combined with the proverbial siddhis, the miraculous powers which nobody has a right to doubt. Even today one may be fortunate enough to meet siddhas in South India in whom all these phenomena are united. These few are living proof that saints of the highest level are not legendary figures.

The reader who now concludes (quite understandably) that despite his desire for the power of a siddha, the practice of yoga is not for Western man, is like a student who abandons the university because he has heard that genius borders on insanity, and he no longer wants to attempt to become a genius.

There are today in India thousands of yogis and hundreds of masters. There are perhaps a few dozen who have realized the highest level of raja yoga, and approximately half a dozen saints on the highest level.

Should we not at least make a beginning and take a few steps toward mastery? For the danger of developing too little yoga and becoming a victim of our inadequate world is far greater than that of becoming an unearthy superman.

RECOMMENDED FOR FURTHER READING

GENERAL

ELIADE, MIRCEA. *Yoga: Immortality and Freedom*. New York, second edition, 1968.

MISHRA, RAMMURTI S. *Fundamentals of Yoga*. New York, 1971.

SHASTRI, HARI PRASAD. *Yoga*. London, 1970.

HATHA YOGA

IYENGAR, B. K. *Light on Yoga*. London, second edition, 1970.

VITHALDAS, YOGI. *The Yoga System of Health*. New York (paper edition), 1957.

RAJA YOGA

MISHRA, RAMMURTI S. *Textbook of Yoga Psychology*. New York, 1971.

WOODS, JAMES HAUGHTON. *The Yoga System of Papanjali*. Delhi, 1966.

HATHA YOGA AND RAJA YOGA

IYANGAR, NIVASA. *The Hatha Yoga Pradipika of Yoga Swami Svatmarama*. Adyar, 1949.

KUVAYALANANDA, SWAMI. *Pranayama*. Bombay, 1966.

SINH, PANCHAM. *Hatha Yoga Pradipika*. Allahabad, 1915.

YOGASHAKTI, PARIVRAJIKA MA. *The Science of Yoga: Commentary on Gherand Samhita*. Bombay, 1966.

INDEX OF YOGA PRACTICES

INDEX OF GENERAL TERMS

bhastrika. A *pranayama*; "the bellows." 87, 92–94, 133

bhramari. A *pranayama* in which the sound of bees is produced. 87, 94

bindu. Period; dot; zero; void; seed; semen. 25, 122, 140–41, 157–59, 166–67, 170, 172, 179–80, 183–84, 187–88

Brahma. One of the gods in the Hindu trinity. See also *Vishnu, Siva.* 46, 57, 60, 85, 165

brahma ananda. The great bliss. 179

brahmacharim. A celibate; a yogi who controls all desires. 64, 133

Brahma granthi. One of the three knots of ignorance. See also *Vishnu granthi* and *Rudra granthi.* 93, 178

Brahman. Supreme power of the universe. 57, 144, 161–62, 185–88

brahmarandra. Crown of the head. 102, 129, 153, 188

caitanya. Pure consciousness. 186

chakras. Wheels; seven centers of energy in the sushumna. 36–37, 47, 49–50, 59, 73, 75, 84, 101–2, 108–9, 128, 131, 141–42, 148–49, 153, 156–57, 165–66, 179–81

chandra. Moon. 75

Charaka Samhita. Standard work of Ayurvedic medicine. 38–40

chaurangi. A *siddha.* 25

daksina. Right side; propitious. 177

dhanurasana. The "bow" posture. 47

dhauti. One of the six *shatkarmas.* To swallow a strip of cloth in order to cleanse the stomach. 81, 83, 85

doshas. The three fundamental terms of Ayurvedic physiology: *vata, pitta,* and *kapha.* 41

gajakarani. To stimulate the nervous system by regurgitating. 84–85

Ganesh. Elephant-headed god with four arms and one tusk; son of Siva and Parvati; god of wisdom who removes obstacles, hence invoked at the beginning of literary works. 23, 165

Ganga. The most sacred river of India; the Ganges. 129–30

ghata. Transition. 178

Gheranda Samhita. A classical yoga text, more recent than Hatha Yoga Pradipika. 49

gomukhasana. The "cow" posture. 43

Gorakshanath. A great *siddha* and founder of a Sivaite sect. 67, 177

196

gunas. The three qualities of Eternal Nature. See also *Rajas, Tamas,* and *Sattva.* 74, 118

guptasana. See *Siddhasana.*

halahala. A mythological poison; the first product to result from the churning of the ocean of milk by the gods and demons. 51–52

ida. The left *nadi.* 56, 75, 104–7, 130, 154, 169, 171

indriyas. The senses. 156, 158, 161

Ishvara. Lord; supreme Deity; stage of complete Self-identification. 134–35

jagra avastha. State of suspended breath; a waking sleep state. 188

jalandhara bandha. The "chinlock" posture. 87, 93, 95, 103–7, 120, 123

japa. Recitation of *mantras.* 32, 144

jivan. Individual soul; empirical soul; germ of life. 116, 121–22

jivanmukta. One liberated in this life. 188

jivatman. Individual self. 145, 182

jnana. Knowledge of the absolute as derived from meditation. 153

jyoti. Light. 130

kala. Time; death; light. 140–41, 166–67, 172, 186–87

kanda. The resting place of kundalini, above the anus. 129, 131

kapala bhati. A mild version of *bhastrika.* 81, 84

kapha. One of the three dominant physiological forces in man, according to the *Ayurveda;* the "fertile water for the play of life"; fluid. 38, 40–41, 50, 80–82, 84, 89–90, 92, 115, 118

karma. The law of universal cause and effect. 65, 112–13, 147–49, 151, 153, 155, 162–63, 168

Keshava. An aspect of *Vishnu.* 165

kevala. Kumbhaka after inhalation. 57–58, 97

khecari mudra. Posture in which the tongue closes the openings (into the throat) of the nasal passage, pharynx, and trachea. 103, 110–14, 118–120, 124, 164, 166–67, 171–72

Krishna. One of the most widely worshipped Hindu deities; teacher of Arjuna in the Bhagavad Gita. 131, 181

kriyavati. Suspension of breath; heat production at crown of head; lifeless body. 78

kukkutasana. The "crow" posture. 44

kumbhaka. The breath suspension between inhalation and exhalation or between exhalation and inhalation; also, a generic term for *pranyama.* 57–58, 63, 69, 73, 75–76, 80, 86–98, 123, 147

kundalini. The "coiled serpent" at the foot of the spine. 44, 49–50, 59–60, 78, 92–93, 97, 101–3, 105–9, 114, 117, 122–24, 127–34, 142, 147–48, 153, 155, 174

kurmasana. The "tortoise" posture. 44–46

laya. Merging; dissolution. 58, 158–63, 177, 181, 184, 186

lingam. Phallic symbol, especially as worshipped in the Sivaite sect. 170–71

Madhava. An aspect of *Vishnu.* 165

mahabandha. The "great" *bandha.* 103, 106–7, 120

mahamudra. The "great" *mudra.* 103, 105–7, 120

maha shunyata. The "great" void. See also *Shunyata.* 180

mahavedha. One of three practices that, when combined, bestow *siddhis.* 103, 107, 120

maithuna. Ritual cohabitation practiced in the cult of *Shaktism.* 127

Mandara. Holy mountain; backbone of the universe. See also *Meru.* 46

manipura chakra. Center in diaphragm region; element of fire. 54–55, 102, 108, 121, 149

mano mani. Deep state of meditation. 119, 144

mantras. Sacred syllables, words, or phrases, recitation and contemplation of which bestows perfection or self-realization; also, the ideal inaudible sounds that make up one aspect of the universe. 32, 71, 109, 130–31, 143–44, 164–66, 168, 172, 176–77, 179, 182, 184, 188

maravaruni. drinking of wine; symbolizes the "flow of nectar from the moon." 146

Matsyendra. Famous yogi and teacher. 25, 42, 124

matsyendrasana. The "fish" posture, first taught by Yogi Matsyendra. 48

maya. The illusory manifestation of the world; the unreality of worldly things. 118, 140

mayurasana. The "peacock" posture. 51, 53

Meru. The mountain supporting the world; symbolizes *sushumna.* See also *Mandara.* 118

moksha. Liberation. See also *Mukti.* 129, 156, 158

mudra. One of ten postures. 63, 68, 101–14, 118–19, 124, 127, 134–35, 147, 165–68 *muktasana.* See *Siddhasana.*

mukti. Liberation. See also *Moksha.* 121

mula bandha. Contraction of the anus muscle. 88, 93, 103, 120, 122–23

muladhara chakra. The lowest *chakra,* at the root of the spinal column; element of earth. 49, 54, 56, 102, 107–8, 121, 131, 134, 142, 148, 157

murccha kumbhaka. A *pranayama.* 87, 95

nabhi granthi. A center in the navel. 89, 93

nada, nadam. Inner sound, primeval sound. See also *Anahat nada.* 64, 80, 98, 122, 140–41, 159, 166–67, 172, 176–88

nadis. Channels in the subtle body. See also *Ida* and *Pingala.* 60, 61, 63, 71–86, 88–89, 90, 92–94, 103–7, 109, 120–21, 123–24, 129–30, 134, 154–55, 165, 169, 171, 178–79

Narayana. An aspect of *Vishnu.* 165

nauli. To draw in the abdominal muscles and rotate them in a churning motion. 81–83

neti. To cleanse the nasal passages by inserting a string or rubber tube into a nostril and pulling it out through the mouth. 81–82, 154

niranjana. Spotless; devoid of *gunas.* 187

nirvana. Extinction of the flame; final emancipation. 24

nishpatti. Perfection; without flaw. 178

niyamas. Observance of ten rules. 32, 127

om. Fundamental sound; *mantra.* 117, 119, 157, 165, 185

paccimasana. A posture in which the legs are held straight and the head touches the knees. 50

padmasana. The "lotus" posture. 53, 58–61, 75, 91

pancagni tapas. The sacrifice of the five fires. 118

paramatman. The Absolute Self. 145, 182, 186

paramesvara. The Divine. 186

paravairagya. A state of samadhi. 186

paricaya. Attainment. 178

Parsis. A Zoroastrian sect; its main community is in Bombay. 11

Parvati. Wife of Lord *Siva.* 156

paschimottasana. See *Paccimasana.* 50

Patanjali. An Indian sage who systematized yogic teachings. 127

pingala. The right *nadi.* 56, 75, 104–7, 130, 154, 169, 171 *pitta.* One of three dominant physiological forces in man, according to the *Ayurveda*; characterized by gall, temperament, heat, fire. 38–41, 49–50, 67, 80, 82, 91–92

plavini. A *pranayama.* 87, 96

prakriti. The Uncaused Cause; Eternal Nature, with three constituents, the *gunas.* Also, the feminine counterpart to *Purusha.* 141, 152

prana. Life force, breath of life. 39, 50–51, 53, 59–60, 62, 72–73, 75–76, 80–81, 84, 88–89, 91–93, 103–8, 114, 117, 120–22, 124, 131–34, 145, 147, 150–59, 171–73, 179, 186

pranayama. Breathing exercise. 37, 63, 73–77, 79–80, 82, 84–86, 89, 92–94, 97, 101, 104, 123, 134, 154, 178, 187

puraka. Inhalation. 87, 97

Puranas. "Old, ancient." Hindu scriptures extolling in legendary form the powers and deeds of positive gods. 109, 114, 164

Purusha. Pure, eternal spirit; the Eternal Conscious Principle, counterpart to Eternal Nature. See also *Prakriti.* 152

Pushkara. One of two mythological isles between which lies the ocean of milk; also, symbol for *sahasrara chakra.* 115

rajas. The second of the three *gunas*; active restlessness. 118

recaka. Exhalation. 87, 97

Rudra granthi. One of the knots that kundalini has to pierce. 93

sadhana. To venerate one's personal deity. 165

sahajoli. To reverse the semen virile in coito. 127, 153

sahasrara chakra. The thousand-petaled lotus on top of the head, where the *kundalini shakti* unites with Lord *Siva,* the Divine Element. 102, 108–9, 115, 128, 134, 153

sahita. Breath in complete balance. 97

samadhi. Deep meditation; the final goal of yoga. 139–49, 155, 158, 168, 171–72, 175, 181–82, 186, 188

samana. One of the five bodily currents. 39

sattva. The highest of the three *gunas.* 74, 118, 157–58, 176

sattvic. Spiritual, pure. 73, 84, 176–77

samskaras. Impressions on consciousness, the seeds of *karma*; activity of the subconscious. 163

savasana. The "dead" posture. 53

Shabara. A *siddha.* 25

Shaka. One of the two mystical isles between which lies the ocean of milk; also symbol for *ajna chakra.* 115

Shakti. The female aspect of the Ultimate Principle; the kinetic agent of consciousness; symbolized as the wife of *Siva.* 25, 128–38, 141, 165, 174–75, 186–87

shakticalana. One of the ten *mudras.* 103, 120

Shaktism. The worship of *Shakti.* 127

shambhavi mudra. Work with *mantras* and *yantras.* 134, 164–75, 177, 183

Shambu. See *Siva.*

shastras. Any sacred book of divine authority; may include the *Vedas.* 117, 124–25, 164, 168, 177

shatkarma. Six ways of physical purification; cleansing of the body. 80–81, 83–84, 121, 154

Siva. One of the gods of the Hindu Trinity; the Destroyer. 23, 25, 52–53, 66, 103, 118–19, 131, 140–41, 144, 166, 172, 177, 185, 187

shunyata. The "great" void. See also *Maha shunyata.* 102

siddha. Possessor of supernatural powers or forces. 23–25, 28, 63–64, 66–67, 83, 103–4, 113, 190

siddhasana. The most important sitting posture. 53–58, 177

siddhi. Supernatural power to perform miracles. 23–25, 27, 68, 80, 86, 103, 106, 118, 124, 127, 133–35, 146, 180

simhasana. The "lion" posture. 53, 62

sirhasana. The headstand. 126

sitali. A *pranayama.* 87, 91–93

sitkari. A *pranayama.* 87, 90, 93

sloka. Terse presentation of esoteric teachings. 50, 58, 64, 109, 113, 126–27, 133, 145, 157, 171

soma. A milky climbing plant (*asclepias acida*), the fermented juice of which is offered in libations to the divinities. Has exhilarating qualities. Also symbolically, the "nectar for the play of life." 40–41, 110–119

Su-meru. See *Meru.*

suryabhedana. A *pranayama.* 75, 87, 89, 93

sushumna. A fine channel in the subtle body; center of the spinal cord; the most important of the *nadis.* 50, 56, 60, 73, 77, 86, 88, 92–93, 97, 102–7, 114, 121–24, 131, 133–34, 147, 152–53, 155, 169, 171–73, 178, 188

sutra. A brief precept or rule. 85, 88, 102

svadhistana chakra. The element of water. 54, 102, 108, 148, 157

svastikasana. A sitting posture. 43

tamas. The third of the three *gunds*; sluggishness. 118

tantra. Rule, ritual. A series of religious texts that emphasize the practice of *japa, mantra,* and other esoteric rituals especially relating to the power of *Shakti.* 103, 140, 168

tapas. Austerities. 31, 67

tat tvam asi. "Thou art that." 32

trataka. To gaze without blinking on a small objec or a candlelight. 81–83

udana. One of the five bodily currents. 39, 85

uddiyana bandha. To draw in the abdominal muscles. 87–88, 93, 103, 120–22, 124, 132

ujjayi. A *pranayama.* 87, 89, 90, 93

unmani avastha. A high meditative state; steadiness of mind; mindless state. 57, 73, 86, 144, 172, 187

upadhis. Attributes that veil and color substance. 186

uttana kurmasana. The "tortoise" posture. 45

vairagya. Dispassion; detachment. 187

vaisheshika. One of the six systems of Indian philosophy. 170

vajrasana. See *Siddhasana.* 55, 132

vajroli. One of the ten *mudras* in which the semen is controlled and reabsorbed into the body. 103, 120, 127, 153

Vasishtha. Rishi; teacher of yoga. 42, 124

vasti. Cleansing of the intestinal tract. 81–82

Vasuki. King of the serpents. 46

vata. One of the three dominant physiological forces in man, according to the *Ayurveda.* 38–41, 50, 71, 80, 89, 92, 118

vayu. Vital breath. 118

Vedas. The most ancient sacred literature of the Hindus. 38, 117, 164

vidya. Ultimate wisdom. 23

viparitakarani. Reversal (of the flow of semen); one of the ten mudras whereby the attributes of the "sun" and the "moon" are reversed; inversion of the body in headstand. 103, 120, 125

virasana. A sitting posture. 43

Vishnu. The second god of the Hindu Trinity; the Unconquerable Preserver. 46, 86

Vishnu granthi. The throat *chakra.* 93, 179

vishudda chakra. The throat center. 54, 102, 108, 117, 123
vyana. One of the five bodily currents. 39

Yama. The king of death; god of death. 106
yamas. Ten rules of conduct; restraints. 31, 56, 75, 127, 133–34
Yamuna. One of the three sacred rivers of India. 129
yantra. A form symbol, contemplation of which leads to self-realization.
     109, 143–44, 146, 164–66, 168, 172, 188